THE BOOK OF

HIGHS

255 Ways to Alter Your Consciousness Without Drugs

EDWARD ROSENFELD

WORKMAN PUBLISHING, NEW YORK

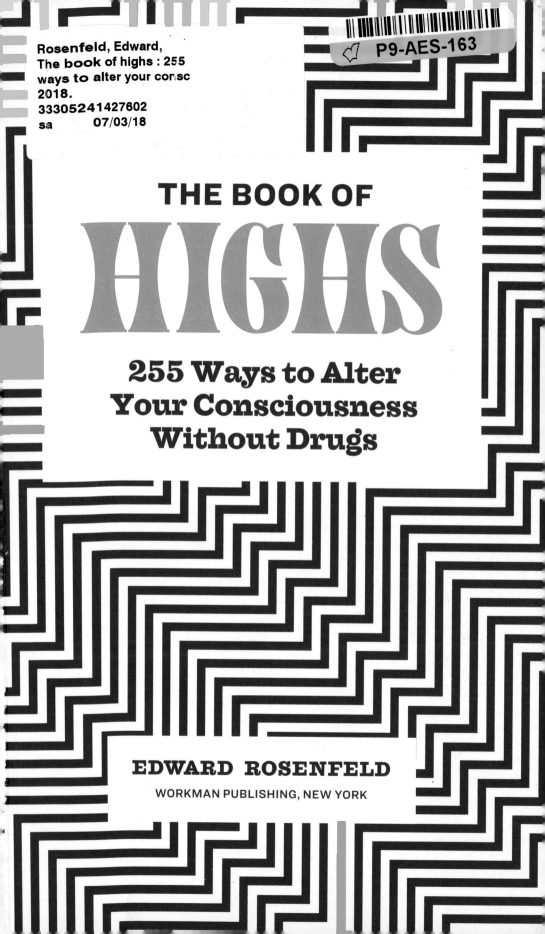

1973: *to D. & G.-W.*
". . . how hard it is
to keep the mind open to surprises!"

—L. L. WHYTE IN *INTERNAL FACTORS IN EVOLUTION*

2018: *To Sylvia, with all my love and affection.*

Originally published in 1973 by Quadrangle/The New York Times Book Co.

Library of Congress Cataloging-in-Publication Data is available.
ISBN 978-0-7611-9387-6

Design by Jean-Marc Troadec
Cover and Interior Illustrations by Nate Duval

Workman books are available at special discounts when purchased in bulk for premiums and sales promotions as well as for fund-raising or educational use. Special editions or book excerpts can also be created to specification. For details, contact the Special Sales Director at the address below, or send an email to specialmarkets@workman.com.

Workman Publishing Co., Inc.
225 Varick Street
New York, NY 10014-4381
workman.com

WORKMAN is a registered trademark of Workman Publishing Co., Inc.

Printed in China
First printing April 2018

10 9 8 7 6 5 4 3 2 1

Acknowledgments

1973: A book of this scope requires the aid of many people. I received much help and guidance. I will attempt to give credit to some; there are numerous others who go unnamed, but not unremembered. The first recognition goes to Frances Cheek, whose idea this was to begin with and who shared that idea so selflessly. My gratitude goes to Bernie Aaronson (and the entire group at the New Jersey Neuropsychiatric Institute), Susan Alexander, Reza Arasteh, Greg Austin, Jeff Berner, Adam Crane, Richie Davidson, Jeremy and the late Rockie Gardiner, Dolly Gattozzi, the late Midge Haber, Harry Hermon, Charles Honorton, the late Mozart and the late Annette Kaufman, Stanley Keleman, Alexandra Kirkland, Stan Krippner, Gay Luce, Eric McLuhan, Ralph Metzner, Marni Miller, the late Gerry Oster, David Padwa, Milo and Celia Perichitch, the late Don Plumley, Ilana Rubenfeld, Pyrrhus Ruches, David Sarlin, the late Steven and Gabriel Simon, Deborah Steinfirst (née Lotus), Klaus von Stutterheim, John Wilcock, Karl Yeargens, and Gene Youngblood.

Without the very special help of others, this work would never have been possible. Elly Greenberg has typed, endured, and given much-needed support. John Brockman has been a helpful and wise friend. Peter Matson's hard work has made this publication possible. The late Bob Masters, Jean Houston, and Bill Wine shared unselfishly of their own work in the area of altered states of consciousness. Charles Tart's *Altered States of Consciousness* has been and continues to be an expansive model.

The late Bennett Shapiro provided help, suggestions, and encouragement, as he did tirelessly for more than two decades. The late Marty Fromm gave me and continues to give me the greatest gift of all: myself.

2018: First thanks go to Melissa Mahoney, who found the original *The Book of Highs* and brought it to her wife, Samantha O'Brien, an editor at Workman. Without Melissa's sharp eyes and sense, this current edition would not have happened. Thanks go to all the crew at Workman, Bruce Tracy, Suzie Bolotin, and Jean-Marc Troadec, but most especially to Sam, an editor without equal. She has guided, inspired, and nourished this book and helped in every way to make it come to a new life. Thanks so much to you, Sam, for your wonderful professionalism, care, and enthusiasm. Thanks to Kenneth Wapner, my literary agent, for his years of work, support, and encouragement.

Other friends and colleagues spared their time, attention, help, and suggestions. Some provided true inspiration, including Sylvia Rosenfeld, Zachary Rosenfeld and Halley, Elinor Greenberg, Gerd Stern, Neal Goldsmith, Stella Resnick, Helen and Tim Atkinson, Frank Spinelli, Tammy Nelson, Gail Woods and Andrzej Nikonorow, Alexandre Tannous, Karen Azlen; they all deserve credit for their help to me and their contributions to this book.

Contents

PART ONE: JUST YOUR SELF

AWARENESS   3

POSITIVE TECHNIQUES   19

NEGATIVE TECHNIQUES 59

FANTASY, SLEEP, DREAMING, AND SEX 79

EVERYDAY LIFE 101

PART TWO: HELP FROM OTHERS

THERAPIES AND MISCELLANEOUS 131

RELIGIONS, MYSTICISM, AND MOVEMENTS 185

PART THREE: DEVICES AND MACHINES

NONELECTRIC   225

ELECTRIC   257

BIOFEEDBACK   281

Getting High and Staying There

by Andrew Weil, author of *The Natural Mind*

A ltered states of consciousness have become so respectable in the past few years that they are now known simply as ASCs—a sure sign that they are in fashion among scientists. Conferences on them are proliferating (one took place recently at the Smithsonian Institution in Washington, D.C.), and month by month ASCs carve out a bigger niche in medical literature. But despite the accumulation of scientific data, we still do not know what it is to be high or the significance of our seeking that state so persistently.

The desire to have peak experiences, to transcend the limitations of ordinary consciousness, operates in all of us. It is so basic that it looks like an inborn drive. Almost as soon as infants learn to sit up, they begin to rock themselves into highs. Later, as young children, they learn to whirl into other states of awareness or hyperventilate out of ordinary reality. Still later they discover drugs.

There has been much talk lately of alternatives to drugs. The present book describes a great many techniques for getting high, none of them making use of drugs. If we could teach people other methods to achieve highs, the drug problem would take on more manageable proportions. But what is wrong with drugs? They certainly work for many people, and, if used with the respect and care they demand, are no more dangerous than many agents in common, legal use in our society.

Some object to drug-induced highs on a puritanical level; it is too easy to get pleasure, let alone religious ecstasy, by swallowing a pill. One ought to work or suffer for that reward. I doubt that any drug user will be convinced by such an argument, especially if pills will do the trick. A more convincing argument borne out by the experience of many users is that drugs sometimes do not do the trick. They may trigger panic states and depressions instead of highs. One can take steps to ensure that a drug experience will be good, but there is always a possibility that unforeseen factors will supervene. The drug itself does not contain the experience it triggers. Highs come from within the individual; they are simply released, or not, by the drug, which always acts in combination with expectations and environment—set and setting.

Drugs reinforce the illusion that highs come from external chemicals when, in fact, they come from the human nervous system. The practical consequence of this illusion-making tendency is that users find it hard to maintain their highs: One always has to come down after a drug high, and the down can be as intense as the up. The user who does not understand this may become dependent on drugs because the easiest way to get out of a low following a high seems to be to take another dose of the drug.

I make no distinction between legal and illegal drugs here. Coffee, an innocent "beverage" in the eyes of many persons, is as dependence-producing as any illegal drug in just this way. The stimulation it provides is offset later by lethargy and mental clouding, usually in the morning. In full-blown coffee addiction a person cannot get going in the morning without his drug, and the more that's consumed, the more the need increases.

Moreover, the more regularly one uses a drug to get high, the less effective it becomes. Many marijuana smokers find that their highs diminish in intensity the more frequently they smoke; chain smokers of weed do not get high at all. Any users of psychedelics, heroin, and amphetamines often look back to their earliest drug experiences as the most pleasureful.

The value of drugs is their ability to trigger important states of consciousness. People who grow up in our materialistic culture may need a drug experience to show them that other modes of consciousness exist. It is notable that the increasingly widespread interest in meditation, intuitive understanding, and spiritual development was spurred by drug-triggered highs giving a glimpse of these other realities. The problem is that drugs cannot be used regularly without losing their effectiveness. They do not maintain highs.

And so there is much searching for other ways of getting high and staying high. Some people say they are looking for more natural methods. But it is difficult to say just what is natural and what is not. Fire walking as practiced in northern Greece may be a terrific high. It is also dangerous when not done correctly; those who try it without proper preparation wind up with badly burned feet. Is it more or less natural than taking mescaline?

The distinction between drug and non-drug methods of getting high might not be very useful, because it is just another product of our current national obsession with drugs. Any technique making use of something material or external to the individual will tend to produce dependence, will tend to lose its effectiveness over time, and will limit one's freedom to get high. Any method requiring things, for example, ties a person to those things—whether they be glowing coals, a biofeedback machine, or tabs of LSD. A better distinction would be between methods that one can use by oneself anytime, anywhere, and methods that require something else. The person who can get high by himself is at a great advantage.

Even if we could convert most of the drug takers in our country into meditators, chanters, or whirling dervishes, I am not certain we would end the dissensions. I think that many people who seem to be anti-drug would be suspicious of any methods used to get out of ordinary awareness. Meditation, for instance, despite all the support of orthodox religion, is often erroneously regarded as an avenue to passive withdrawal from the world and would doubtless stir up much opposition if it were practiced openly on a larger scale. To the rational, straight side of our consciousness, the search for better highs may look like simple hedonism and a shirking of all responsibility.

No doubt some persons are just out for new thrills and pleasures. But the drive to get high that appears in earliest infancy cannot be there for no reason at all; it is too basic a need. And many nonordinary experiences are not pleasureful—they are powerful, different, strange, even terrifying. Still, we call them "highs" because somehow they seem fraught with positive potential and the capacity to change us for the better.

If we look over an extensive catalog of methods for getting high, one common trait stands out: They all are techniques of focusing awareness, of shaking us out of habitual modes of perception and getting us to concentrate on something, whether a sound, a sight, or an unusual sensation. Possibly, what we call a high is simply the experience of focused consciousness, even if the focus is on something we would normally consider painful or unpleasant. And possibly, when our ordinary consciousness is focused on anything, we can become aware of what is ordinarily unconsciously perceived: our internal organs, for example, or other persons' minds or even things beyond ordinary time and space.

Concentration is the key. In "normal" states of mind, our conscious energies are scattered. Our attention wanders aimlessly from thought to thought to external sensations to internal sensations to the past to the future to snatches of tunes to hopes and fears to images to objects. Nearly all systems of meditation require preliminary practice at concentration, at stilling the restlessness of the ever-observing mind. Meditation is nothing other than directed concentration. Concentration is power.

Sometimes we enter states of concentration spontaneously, without making any efforts. An intensely pleasureful, painful, or unusual stimulus can draw our single-minded attention so completely that we simply find ourselves in an altered state of consciousness. All of us have the capacity to enter these states, and all of us probably spend time in them even if we are not aware of it. And the states are natural whether the means used to achieve them are peculiar or not. In this sense it is natural to be high and natural to want to be high.

In fact, being high might be the most natural condition of all. The euphoria of a state of focused awareness is almost always accompanied by a conviction that it is the way things are "supposed to be." Instead of learning to get high, we may have to unlearn not being high; by ridding ourselves of the learned habits of worrying, fearing, and scattering mental energy, we get down to that core feeling of joyful transcendence that is the basic state of the human nervous system.

Far from leading to withdrawal from the world, meditation and other self-reliant methods of getting high tend to make us better able to function in ordinary reality. The better we get at getting high and staying there, the more we integrate the conscious and unconscious spheres of our mental life. This integration is the key to wholeness (health) of body and mind.

We are caught up in a fever of experimentation with methods of changing consciousness, much of it generated by the young. There will be much wasted effort, some casualties. But out of it all will come a generation that will know how to use its consciousness more and more fully—a generation that can build a truly high society.

A. W.

TUCSON, ARIZONA

MARCH, 1973

Preface

"If the doors of perception were cleansed every thing would appear to man as it is, Infinite. For man has closed himself up, till he sees all things thro' narrow chinks of his cavern."

—WILLIAM BLAKE, THE MARRIAGE OF HEAVEN AND HELL

Inspired by Blake, Aldous Huxley described his experiences with altered states of consciousness in his book *The Doors of Perception* (from which the rock group the Doors took their name). The experiences Huxley wrote about in that book, and in his other works, were a result of taking psychedelics. Following Blake's poetic observation, Huxley realized, while in an altered state of awareness, that the brain basically behaves as a reducing valve, acting as a filter of Blake's Infinite: "What comes out at the other end is a measly trickle of the kind of consciousness which will help us to stay alive on the surface of this particular planet." In other words, our brains and bodies try to regulate the full power of our consciousness. But occasionally widening this valve, as humans have sought to do since the beginning of recorded history, gives us a glimpse into the Infinite.

The profound experiences that Blake and Huxley so eloquently and poetically express are vital to me and have enhanced me in living a full life. When laws were being enacted in the 1960s to make sure that psychedelic drugs were made illegal, I was troubled, outraged, and motivated to take action. When I considered the legislation seeking to curtail access to and use of psychedelics, I thought: *They can outlaw drugs, but CONSCIOUSNESS CANNOT BE OUTLAWED! Not even altered states of consciousness!* I believed by assembling and compiling into book form at least a short list of ways to get high without drugs, I could make sure that these extraordinary states of being would be available to all. I published this compilation as *The Book of Highs* in 1973.

In the decades since, much has changed in the ways we get high and how we treat altered states. After decades of being described as unworthy of research, psychedelics are, once again, being investigated and experimented with in order to discern their applicability to many important aspects of life, such as end-of-life anxiety and post-traumatic stress disorders. And the general condition of altered states of consciousness is now the subject and focus of much new attention. Consider the consciousness-hacking movement, which focuses on how technology can help us reach altered states (for examples, see this book's entries on the Mutual Wave Machine and exciting advancements in Biofeedback). As someone wrote me recently: "We're living in the golden age of getting high—there's no better time for a revised edition of your book."

I welcomed the opportunity to extend and expand *The Book of Highs*, with connections to modern technology like virtual reality, video games, and the ever-expanding world of the web. While the original book directed readers to film archives and vinyl records, this new edition offers YouTube and Spotify playlists with recordings, chants, films, and animated illusions. So much is available to all of us now, we need only seek out our passions and what we want to know, and infinite resources are there for us to use and enjoy. Even as pernicious drug laws are revamped, changed, and rescinded, the myriad approaches to getting high deserve more scrutiny, focus, and exploration. New highs will be born anew in the future, as people seek adventures in consciousness and being. Here's hoping this book will inform, delight, and serve many.

—EDWARD ROSENFELD, APRIL 2018

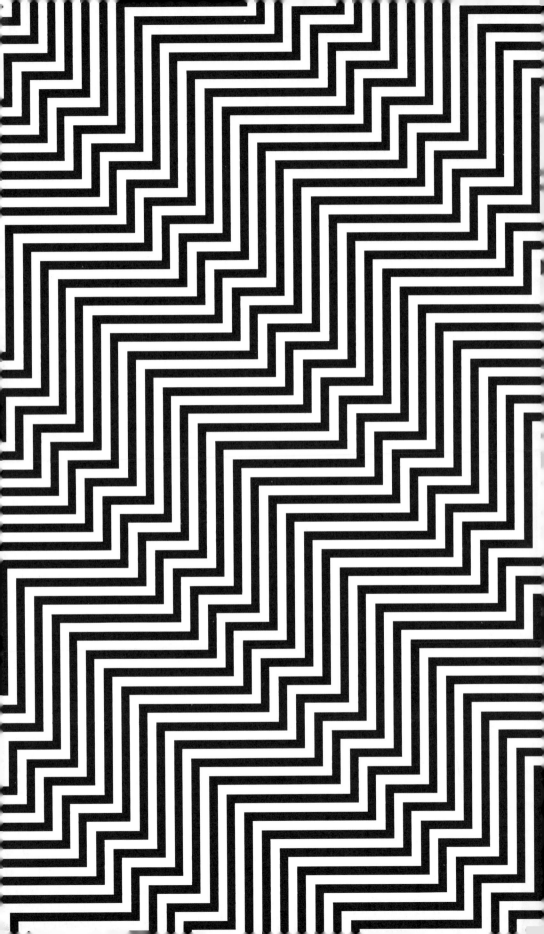

PART ONE
JUST YOUR SELF

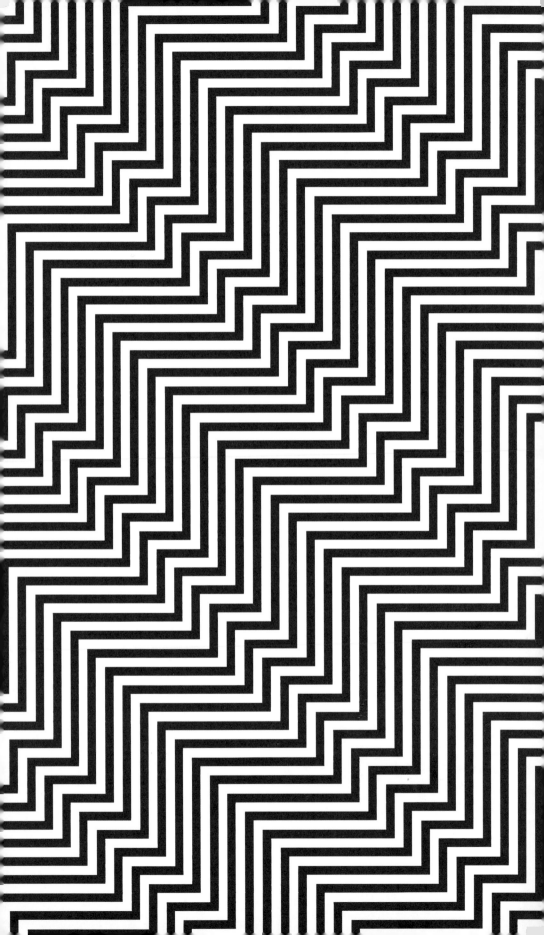

CHAPTER 1

AWARENESS

1 Concentration

Focusing and staying with it.

The development of concentration—that is, our ability to direct our attention at will—is germane to many of the techniques and methods described in this book. We usually go through our days paying little attention to our environment. It is only occasionally that we actually "take in" a particular object, image, thought, or person. We fail, almost always, to concentrate.

Concentration means learning to focus; it means training ourselves, through practice, to "stay with" the object of our attention despite distraction; it means staying with a subject and "mastering" our relationship with the subject. (This does not mean mastering the subject! Real concentration indicates a relationship of equality, an I-Thou relationship with the subject.)

Our attention should be directed toward the field, both interior and exterior, of our environment. That field is made up of Gestalten—literally, configurations or patterns. In order for these configurations to become meaningful, part of the pattern serves as background so that another part of it will stand out as the foreground. Life itself is a continuum of such changing and transforming figure-ground interactions.

To concentrate means to establish a clear Gestalt, so that the foreground figure stands predominant—clear of the background. Being able to stay with the figure is concentration. Powers of concentration can be developed through practice. Pick a thought, idea, object, and/or person, and stay with it. Devote your attention to it. This is surprisingly difficult. You will generally notice how your attention wanders. Bring the subject back into focus, and stay with it. Remember, the process is more important than the subject of concentration.

Try an experiment: concentrate on one of your fingertips. Carefully examine the lines that are etched there. Treat them as though they were a maze, and choose a beginning and end. Don't resist when your attention fades; stay with your experience. Find out what happens to your concentration when it wanders.

Further Resources

Christmas Humphreys's book *Concentration and Meditation* is a good general introduction. The first four exercises in *Gestalt Therapy* by Frederick S. Perls, Ralph Hefferline, and Paul Goodman show how to go about concentrating, from the phenomenological point of view. Other aids may be found in this book under Meditation (No. 14), Yoga (No. 149), and Buddhism (No. 157).

• •

2 Self-awareness

Experience your *self*.

This section's entries all deal with self-awareness. Not yourself, but your *self*. Anything that alters consciousness, with or without drugs, provides the potential for increased awareness of your self.

Ride in a car at 60 mph. It seems quite fast at the beginning. Maintain a speed of 60. Your awareness of it will slowly diminish. Then slow down to 30 mph and accelerate back up to 60. Another way to increase awareness of the constant 60 mph speed is to change what you see. Instead of looking ahead onto the road unfolding before you, look down at the road directly beneath. The "slowness" of 60 mph quickly disappears.

So it is with your self. When we continue our usual lifestyles, repeating the same actions over and over, getting tied into habits, not paying attention to either the fine details or the overall general patterns and trends of existence, we don't notice who is *living* the life. Pay attention, concentrate, tune in to the meaning of your existence. Your life is *real*. Experience yourself as an animal, part of the species, a biological phenomenon filled with cells and systems and organs, rhythmically crawling, walking, running, rolling, and flying around the surface of the planet. Become ever more aware of how fantastic your universe-presence is. William Blake said, "If the doors of perception were cleansed every thing would appear to man as it is, infinite." As it is.

Further Resources

The methods, techniques, and approaches discussed in this book are meant to be helpful. I have found a combination of phenomenology, existentialism, altered states of consciousness, Zen Buddhism, Gestalt therapy, and planetary awareness to be helpful. Other combinations may help you. Different strokes for different folks.

3 Philosophical awareness

"Perseverance furthers."

Philosophy may be thought of as speculative inquiry into our nature. Through philosophical awareness we focus our attention on the questions and problems brought about by the "facts" of our existence; through philosophical awareness we may be able to effect a relationship with certain manifestations of our lives.

What is it to be alive?

What is the meaning of life?

Who am I?

Am I real?

Who are you?

What is the world (Earth)? Solar system? Galaxy? Universe?

What is knowledge?

One of the major problems in dealing with questions like these is our language. To answer the question: "What is the meaning of life?" an answer must be constructed that begins: "The meaning of life is . . ." Because our language reflects our reality, what we are able to *describe* can circumscribe what we are able to *experience*.

Such are the traps that we encounter in attempting to cultivate philosophical awareness. The experience of the Austrian philosopher Ludwig Wittgenstein (1889–1951) is a profound example of some of the difficulties of philosophical thought. His two major published works contradict each other. The first, *Tractatus Logico-Philosophicus* (1921), provides a general and ultimate philosophical theory. His second work, *Philosophical Investigations* (published posthumously in 1953), rejects any such general theory and examines many individual cases without general comment. As he wrote: "In philosophy we do not draw conclusions . . . philosophy only states what everyone admits."

The *attempt* to reach conclusions in philosophy, though often frustrating and contradictory, can be liberating. The *I Ching* says: "Perseverance furthers." See where your limits and contradictions lie. Can you transcend them through thought? Ponder, persevere.

Further Resources

Philosophers of the West are covered in Bertrand Russell's *A History of Western Philosophy.* Many Eastern philosophies are referred to later in this volume. Contemporary philosophical trends are reviewed in the works of Colin Wilson, in *The Age of Complexity* by Herbert Kohl, and in Susanne Langer's *Philosophy in a New Key.*

· ·

4 Sensory awareness

You do not *have* senses; you *are* your senses.

We receive information from and about our environment through our senses. The primary senses are:

Vision (eyes)
Hearing (ears)
Smell (nose)
Taste (tongue, mouth, and nose)
Touch (skin and tongue)

Our senses continually process an amazing amount of information. Here again, the Gestalt theory of figure-ground formation is important to our understanding. When we open our eyes we observe and focus our visual attention on one subject. The other objects in that same visual field form the background against which that figure stands out.

There are many different methods, techniques, and exercises that can help us to develop our sensory awareness.

The best way to develop the senses is to find out what it's like to live without them. This is called *sensory deprivation.* Sight lends itself to this experiment best. Select an environment that you know very well—your house, your room, or someplace equally familiar. Close your eyes or wear a blindfold, and sightlessly examine your environment. Pay attention to those senses you use when you cannot see. You will depend on your sense of touch to feel your way around; you may also use your sense of smell*; you will hear sounds to which you rarely pay conscious attention.

Another experiment is to isolate a block of time, say five minutes, during which you will be performing some everyday task or activity (changing your clothes, going to the bathroom, coming home from work, etc.). Pay careful attention to everything that you touch during this period. If you are wearing clothing, examine every point and surface where your skin and clothing touch. Do not *do* anything with your observations. Stay with what you are feeling.

Now try the same experiment employing the senses of smell and hearing.

We usually associate tasting with food, but there are many other possibilities. We always have some taste in our mouths: our own saliva, pens, glasses, etc. Try paying attention to them and pay special attention to the way utensils such as saucers, bowls, and silverware affect the taste of food with their own separate tastes.

You might select a variety of herbs to taste—parsley, sage, rosemary, thyme—and spend five minutes with each. Taste and stay with the experience of salt, butter, oil, and ketchup. Try butter and caraway seeds, or make up concoctions of your own.

Bernard Gunther developed techniques which attempt to re-establish contact with sensory experience, to quiet compulsive and habitual thought, to end chronic tension, and to help free trapped potential and awareness. Gunther describes two of these exercises:

> Blind Shower: Step in the shower and close your eyes. Shampoo your hair. Soap your whole body. Rinse and dry yourself completely before you open your eyes.

> Silent Meal: Share a meal with someone or with a group without talking. Listen to sounds; smell, taste, touch, see, feel. Eat some of the meal with your eyes closed. Variations: (1) Eat part of or the whole meal with your hands. (2) Serve one dish, like ice cream or yogurt, that must be eaten without utensils or the use of the hands.

By experiencing your senses, rather than possessing them, you will revitalize your sensory awareness. You do not *have* senses; you *are* your senses.

Other species rely heavily on smell for navigation: Unless the mazes used for lab rats are thoroughly sterilized, the rats smell their way through them.

Further Resources

A good introduction to sensory work is provided in the article "Report on Work in Sensory Awareness and Total Functioning" by Charlotte Selver and Charles V. W. Brooks, which appears in Herbert Otto's *Explorations in Human Potentialities.* Exercises 6 and 13 in *Gestalt Therapy* by Perls et al., can be helpful. Gunther's techniques for opening up new channels of sensory awareness are described in *Sense Relaxation* and *What to Do Until the Messiah Comes.* Also see *Joy* by William Schutz and the Sensory Awareness Foundation (sensoryawareness.org).

· ·

5 Biological awareness

What are we made of?

We often fail to remember that we are an animal species. Our powers of communication have become so great and vast that we have forgotten how recently we left the trees. What is necessary is perspective. A trip to the zoo or, better, a weaponless eco-friendly safari, will remind us that we are biologically linked to the species on our planet. Better organized than some, less peaceful than most, lacking in spontaneity yet exceedingly intelligent—still, we are animals. We are MEAT. We are flesh and cells and neurons and blood, organs and bone and marrow. We are hair and muscle and teeth and secretion and waste. What are we made of? What are we made from? How do we keep making?

Reduce experience to the cellular level. Learn about cells and *be* your cells; rather, be *cells.* Be invisible!

Feel your needs, feel your revulsions. Experience your levels and all of your strata. Flow like blood; leap and charge like a nerve impulse across a synapse.

Imagine anthropologists from another world observing and visiting us. What might they find? What words would they use to describe us?

Further Resources

For the topological and geological groundwork consult Gray's *Anatomy* and Royce's *Surface Anatomy.* For "meat" considerations see Michael McClure's *Meat Science Essays.* An extraterrestrial anthropological report is contained in Arthur C. Clarke's *Report on Planet Three.* For cellular awareness, see Kees Bokes's *Cosmic View.*

6 Visceral awareness

Know your body. Be a body.

W e are systems, and we take totally for granted the fact that hundreds of thousands of "parts" are acting synergistically to keep us in action. Our systems include:

the skeletal

the muscular

the sensory

the circulatory

the respiratory

the gastrointestinal

the genitourinary

the endocrine

the nervous

Glands, networks, and organs all work cooperatively for your maintenance. All operate without your instructions and without your knowledge.

To get in touch with how your insides work, find out what *makes* them work. Find out as much as possible through your own concentration. Listen for the pumping of your heart. Zero in on the heat of your liver. Pay attention to the contractions of your stomach. Feel the changes in tension as your urine leaves your bladder.

Know your body.

Be a body.

Further Resources

F or some assistance in this area see the resources for Nos. 242–245.

. . . .

7 Rhythmic and cyclical awareness

Become aware of all your bodily rhythms.

The rhythms and cycles that we experience in our lives are part of a delicate universal balance. Most of our changes, like sleeping, waking, becoming hungry, eating, etc., are connected to the permutations in our solar system, especially those involved in the relationship between the earth, the sun, and moon. Other rhythms include those influenced by cosmic rays, electromagnetic fields, gravity, and planetary motion. The most important rhythm, the most meaningful cycle on earth, is the circadian or daily rhythm. The word *circadian* comes from the Latin *circa dies*—about a day. There are two daily cycles: the solar day, which has 24 hours, and the lunar day, which has 24.8 hours.

Rhythms and cycles direct your sleep and dreams. They vary your body temperature as much as two degrees during each circadian cycle. Your blood, blood sugar, urine, hormones, energy, and stress all flow to prescribed rhythms.

Sense and feel your rhythmic cycles, stay in touch with them. Be your rhythms. Feel your body temperature at 99 degrees Fahrenheit, at the peak of your daily cycle. Know that when you sleep your temperature is near 97 degrees Fahrenheit.

The adrenal hormones function so that dinner has a more pronounced aroma than lunch or breakfast. Noises sound louder at night, and bright lights are easier to tolerate after you've slept. As the day progresses, your steroid levels decrease and your ability to make sensory discriminations diminishes.

The moon controls many aspects of life. The tides obey the pull of the moon, as do the menstrual cycles of women. At the beginning of this moon cycle there is a buildup of tension as well as an increase in bodily fluids. After the periodic cycle is complete, there is a release from this tension and a sense of well-being.

Police have noted that crimes of violence and passion increase during the full moon and the new moon.

Energy levels also change with the seasons. Tune in to your body's storing and spending of energy. When you are depressed, examine your sleep cycle; check your internal clock. Become aware of all your bodily rhythms.

Further Resources

See Gay Gaer Luce's *Body Time* and R. Ward's *The Living Clocks.* There is also a vast array of apps available for tracking your body's cycles, particularly for women's menstruation, such as Clue (helloclue.com) or Planned Parenthood's Spot On (spotontracker.org).

. . . .

8 Planetary awareness

Contemplating our extraordinary home of Earth.

It's easy to forget that we are living on the surface of a planet. We cannot truly feel the immense pull of gravity, we cannot see or feel the Earth spin (see Culturally based visual illusions, No. 28), we may never experience parts of our far-reaching, diverse globe firsthand (oceans, rainforests, deserts).

Take a moment to contemplate our extraordinary home: We live in a small envelope of protective (and destructive) gases that surrounds the outer surface of a medium-size planet. That supportive envelope also maintains a variety of vegetables and minerals which in turn maintain us in our universe. The key to this system, as to all systems in the universe, is the relative transformation of energy. Prior to humankind's acute posttribal awareness of energy, we had no problem maintaining a balanced relationship with the planet's energy transformations. But since the beginning of urban culture, the rapidly expanding development of the modern world has upset the balance of many Earth systems.

Unfortunately, being aware of our planet is now intertwined with being aware of its destruction. We have destroyed the old ecology; it will never live again. We are creating, without conscious ecological direction, a new environmental system that will eventually destroy our species, as global warming demonstrates on a near-daily basis. Awareness of climate change, species extinction, and other dangerous trends has grown and spread in the twenty-first century, and agreements between nations have been reached to achieve changes. But there's still so much more that needs to be done.

If humanity is to survive, a new, consciously created, anticipated, participatory, planetary ecology must be achieved, for it has become impossible to "return" to the old Earth ecology. Many issues are bound up in domains that seem far from the environment and ecology, like the complications from installed base, wealth aggregation, and political disfunction.

Planet Earth has enough energy at hand, through wind, waves, the Sun, and other clean-energy approaches to satisfy global energy needs. But weaning the planet from the bad energy extraction habits of the past is difficult and many needed changes would threaten the 1 percent of the planet's population who control much of Earth's wealth. Changing policy is difficult, especially on a global basis. When we all face grave, life-threatening issues, however, we have a history of coming up with workable solutions. The control of the use of nuclear weapons since World War II is, so far, a good and inspiring example of what can be done to deal with imminent threats. Other solutions, which may seem radical or even over the top, like E. O. Wilson's suggestion to reserve a large fraction of the planet's surface in its wildness, may point us all in the directions in which we will have to go to continue to enjoy ecological/planetary awareness and life on Earth.

As complex and busy as our daily lives are, just contemplating our animal life on the surface of this awesome and beautiful planet, spinning through the universe, can provide an altered state of awareness, right now! Take a moment to remember all the beautiful details of the home we call Earth and its place in the vast universe. Your life depends on it.

Further Resources

All of the works of Buckminster Fuller and John McHale are essential in this area. Especially helpful are the World Design Science Decade Documents (1–6). The best introduction to current thought in ecology is *The Subversive Science,* edited by Paul Shepard and Daniel McKinley. Boeke's *Cosmic View* covers the entire universe, macrocosmically and microcosmically, in forty simple but wonderfully effective pictures. For a view of the ecological situation under our feet see Rudolf Geiger's *The Climate Near the Ground.* Barry Commoner reviews contemporary problems of ecology and speaks forcefully about their solutions in *The Closing Circle.* For a contemporary take on climate and planetary awareness, see Elizabeth Kolbert's *The Sixth Extinction.*

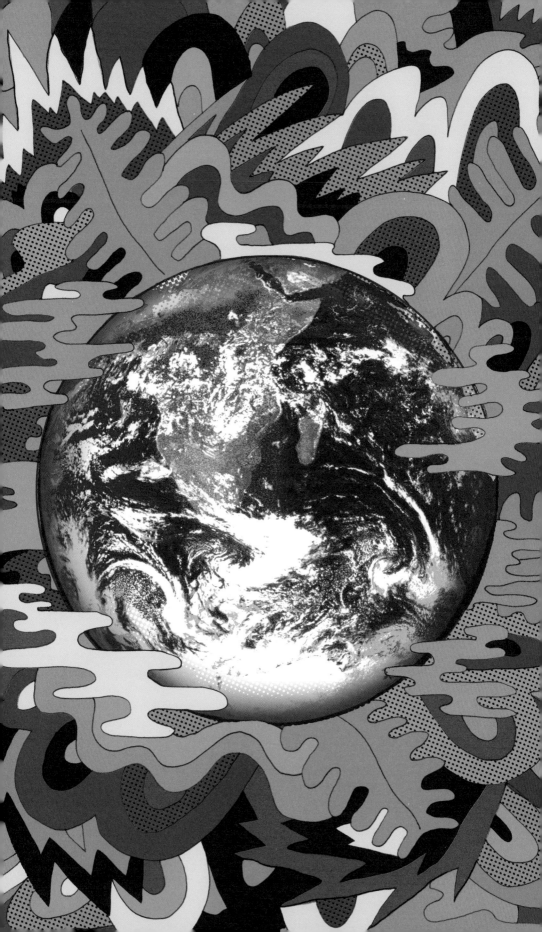

· ·

9 Short-lived phenomena

Eruptions, earthquakes, tsunamis, and more.

Mice plagues, lost tribes, black snow, bird irruptions, meteorite finds, volcanic eruptions, tsunamis, earthquakes, tornadoes, hurricanes, beached whales, fireballs, butterfly invasions, and comets are all short-lived phenomena.

The appearance and experience of such phenomena have the propensity to shake you up and jolt you out of your normal state of consciousness. Anyone who has witnessed, live, one of these kinds of events can attest to their intensity and mind- and body-altering capacities.

Further Resources

Information on such occurrences was once reported by the Smithsonian Institution's Center for Short-Lived Phenomena. The Smithsonian archives (siarchives.si.edu/blog) provides a brief history of the center. Apparently, after some restructuring CSLP became the Scientific Event Alert Network (SEAN), and SEAN went on to become the Global Volcanism Program, which is based at the National Museum of Natural History.

· ·

10 Semantic awareness

The limits of my language are the limits of my world. — LUDWIG WITTGENSTEIN

When we communicate our ideas, thoughts, and opinions to each other, our words carry powerful messages. These messages may not be communicated through pronunciation or grammatical structure; but they are always present in *how* we say what we say. A good example of this is the salutation "Hi, slowpoke!" jokingly spoken by the jealous observer to the runner just finishing a workout. Even though it *seems* to have been said in jest, here the message is in the literal meaning of the words. The speaker has revealed his secret jealousy.

Other indicators of semantic awareness are attention to whether our language is general or specific; whether it judges or shows objectivity; and whether the attitude contained in our words shows an open or a closed stance.

A good experiment is to set aside one day for taking everything said to you exactly at face value. Even when people are kidding you, respond as though they are giving you a sermon. If someone says something sarcastic or facetious, treat it as though they had shared a most profound insight with you. The point of this experiment is to show that people almost *always* say exactly what they mean, even when they conceal it in sarcasm or facetiousness.

Another good experiment is to set aside a day in which you take pains to make sure every sentence you speak is a complete one. Every sentence you hear should also be complete. If someone says something to you in an incomplete sentence, take it upon yourself to finish it.

Still another language game is to be aware of every exaggeration, every disproportionate allusion, and every overstatement. Remember that we mean what we say, and we are what we say and how we say it.

Further Resources

The works of Ludwig Wittgenstein, though difficult, are among the most intense and thorough considerations of language that we have. A good general introduction is *The Meaning of Meaning* by C. K. Ogden and I. A. Richards. *Science and Sanity* by Alfred Korzybski is more specific and outlines a method of awareness, General semantics (see No. 114). Benjamin Lee Whorf's *Language, Thought, and Reality* examines man's behavior and view of reality as a function of his language.

• •

11 Extraspecies communication

Our attempts to communicate with other species, animal and alien, reveal much about ourselves.

If science-fiction fantasy became the science-fact reality and we were the subjects of a visitation by another species with whom we could establish communication, would we be ready? Would we know what to say or how to say it? Of course we would know how to ask *them* who they were, what their purpose was, and so on. But who are we? What is our purpose?

Information is a measure of one's freedom of choice when one selects a message.
—WARREN WEAVER

John Lilly conducted much research in the field of extraspecies communication. In his work with dolphins he may have opened the way for communication with a nonhuman, intelligent species right here on Earth. In considering extraspecies, extraplanetary communications, Lilly concluded:

> With the current picture as it is, I would advise any being greater or lesser than we are not to contact us. In our present state of development, we are still unsuitably organized and unsuitably educated to make contact.

Sometimes our attempts to communicate with other species reveals much about our own. Consider the Voyager Golden Record, a program led by Carl Sagan, which selected the best recordings to represent humanity and launched them into space. On the record: greetings in fifty-five languages, classical music, the sounds of thunder and a kiss, the song "Johnny B. Goode," and more.

Further Resources

See John Lilly's *Man and Dolphin* and *The Mind of the Dolphin*. And, of course, lots of science fiction. Arthur C. Clarke's *Childhood's End* and Ted Chiang's "Story of Your Life" (adapted into the movie *Arrival*) come immediately to mind. Information about the Golden Record can be found on NASA's website (voyager.jpl.nasa.gov). Several of its recordings are included on the *Book of Highs* Spotify playlist.

· ·

12 Cultural awareness

One must know one's culture to rise above it.

Cultural assimilation is important for transcendence. If you don't know your own culture, it becomes very difficult to rise above it, to see through the cultural manipulations that keep us in a state of stagnation.

If changes from outside your culture are to be brought to bear with authority and meaning, a firm grounding and understanding of your own cultural manifestations are required. Being able to experience your culture fully indicates a readiness for new insights and developments.

Altered states of consciousness bring new awareness and often insights that seem to tap a universal core of species experience, a collective unconscious. Without knowledge of one's culture—behaviors, language, beliefs—a person will face great difficulty in sharing these newfound insights with their acquaintances. For example, a student may tell his parents that they and he are really God, that we are all one. But since they have no background in relating to this idea, they will probably be hostile to it. The student's approach, proceeding without clues indicating receptivity, indicates his cultural insensitivity. Cultural assimilation helps one to bring it all home in subtle and meaningful ways.

Re-culturation contributes to re-integration and happens whenever the individual has assimilated his own culture; it then becomes a step toward the next re-birth.
—A. REZA ARASTEH, SCHOLAR WHO COMBINED WESTERN PSYCHOLOGY AND SUFISM

Free men obey the rules which they themselves have made.
—ALFRED NORTH WHITEHEAD, MATHEMATICIAN AND PHILOSOPHER

· ·

13 Awareness of others

Heaven is other people.

Though it often seems that our skin envelopes shut us in, make us ultimately untouchable, we are not alone. Even on the most mundane level, this is obvious. Sartre said, "Hell is other people." Heaven is other people, too. We are other people.

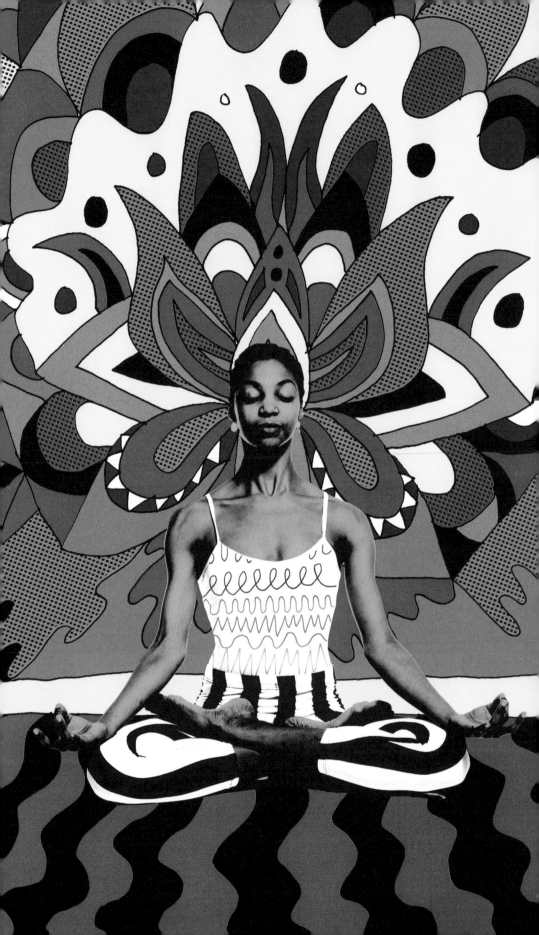

CHAPTER 2

POSITIVE TECHNIQUES

14 Meditation

Meditation is essentially:
sitting quietly, doing nothing;

or, perhaps better:
quietly, doing no-thing, here/now.

The fundamentals of all meditation are centered in your self, wherever you may be—STILL, ON THE MOVE, OR DOING NOTHING BUT THAT WHICH YOU ARE DOING AT THAT MOMENT.

Make or do? How do you do other than do?
—JOHN BROCKMAN

A simple sitting meditation procedure is described below. There are many to fit different temperaments. Try out as many as you can and pick the one that suits you best.

Find a place where you won't be disturbed, a comfortable spot where you will be able to sit for at least thirty minutes. Many believe that more difficult, arduous positions, like the crossed legs of the full- and half-lotus are more helpful during meditation. (In full-lotus, one sits with the legs crossed so that the outside of the right foot rests on the inside of the left thigh and the outside of the left foot rests on the inside of the right thigh. In half-lotus only one foot is placed on one thigh, with the other leg crossed beneath.) Others have found that meditation can be accomplished proficiently even while sitting in a chair. It is important to keep the spine straight, but not rigid, and perpendicular to the floor.

After getting into this posture, fold your hands in your lap. You might find that your meditation will be enhanced if, when putting your hands in your lap, you place your palms upward. Many religious leaders believe that the position with the palms up is one of great receptivity, allowing energy to enter the person.

Once this position is attained and you feel comfortable, sit quietly for about fifteen or twenty minutes. Later, when you have had more experience, you might find that half-hour sitting periods are preferable. When you meditate, do not close your eyes; it becomes very easy to drift off to sleep. Keep them open and let your gaze fall a few feet in front of you. Fix on a spot but do not stare; rather, let the eyes stop there without really looking. With your eyes on this spot, direct your vision inward.

What is most interesting in meditation is the state of being that can develop: a quality of clear attention and a great ability to focus and concentrate. To develop these qualities, some masters assign a mantra, or group of sacred syllables, to a meditator. The meditator is instructed to concentrate on his mantra as the center of his focusing.

In the Zen school, meditation begins by focusing on breathing. First, breaths are counted on the exhalation. Later, inhalations are counted, and still later, both are noted. After this has been accomplished one might be told to watch breaths flowing in and out of their body, but not to count them. Still later, a Zen master might assign a *koan*, or problem, as the focus of meditation.

A very difficult but rewarding form of meditation is the meditation on nothing, or no-thing. This brings about an encounter with paradox. If the object of meditation is nothing and you reach this object, recognition that you have arrived at nothing will constitute something, won't it? Perhaps nothing will become no-other-thing-but-this, the latter being what is at the center of consciousness in the here and now. Meditation can lead to the experience of that place.

Further Resources

Some very enlightening recent texts on meditation include Thich Nhat Hanh's Mindfulness Essentials series, Daniel Siegel's *Mind: A Journey to the Heart of Being Human,* and Sharon Salzberg's *Real Happiness* and *Real Happiness at Work.* To that list I would add Christmas Humphreys's *Concentration and Meditation,* Charles Luk's *Secrets of Chinese Meditation,* Kapleau's *Three Pillars of Zen,* Chogyam Trungpa's *Meditation in Action,* Maharishi Mahesh Yogi's *The Science of Being and the Art of Living,* and Paul Reps's delightful *Ten Ways to Meditate.* Also see resources for some of the Religions and Mysticism entries.

. . . .

15 Prolonged observation

Staring and staying with it.

This is one of the easiest ways to alter consciousness without taking drugs. It requires only concentration, yourself, and an object. The basic method for turning on through prolonged observation is: STAY WITH IT!

Although visual experience is described, one can transpose this same technique to fit the other senses. Select something; say, a flower. Go (with the flower) where you can relax and where you won't be disturbed or distracted. Get into a frame of mind so that you will attend only to the flower. Hold it about six inches in front of your eyes or as close as necessary to bring it into sharp focus. Look at the flower. STAY WITH IT! Some people experience nothing for a couple of minutes. Try not to blink. Of course you will have to, but try to make each uninterrupted period of contact between you and the flower last as long as possible. Try to move as little as possible and STAY WITH IT!

After five minutes you will have noticed the changes that both the flower and the background have gone through. The boundary where the flower ends and the background begins will start to blur. The edges of surrounding objects will begin to look funny and fuzzy. With intense concentration faces might appear in the flower; movements that don't exist might be noticed. This experience is very similar to the altered perception reported by people who have taken psychedelic drugs.

You can use anything for your object. A flower is small and provides lots of background. A piece of white paper provides a large, eye-filling field that generally flows and undulates after a few moments. Other possibilities abound in your everyday environment. Two favorites are fingerprints and your own mirror image. Using another person in this exercise is also interesting. One of the curious things about this technique is the fact that it often occurs spontaneously with people who are in positions where prolonged observation is inevitable—sentry duty and the watch on a ship.

. . . .

16 Spinning

Whirl like a dervish.

"Prayer has a form, a sound, and a physical reality," writes Rumi, the Persian Sufi poet.

The universe is in *all* directions.

Spinning around is guaranteed to turn you on. It is easy to do and, when done correctly, as children do it, spinning is safe.

It is better to spin out of doors. Find a beautiful place where the ground is soft enough to fall on.

Stand still. Start spinning. Feel the beat of your heart. Spin around and around. Spin in a counterclockwise direction, even if you are left-handed. Use one foot as the pusher and the other as the balance. The Sufi whirling dervishes hold their arms out like wings, with the fingers of their right hands pointing up to the sky to receive energy and grace and the palms of their left hands pointing down to the earth, as a means of dispensing their divine gifts to mankind.

Use your heart to generate a mystical current, as the Sufis do when they spin for their master.

If you fall down, get back up and keep spinning. If you can't keep spinning, stop. The world will keep spinning around you.

Around and around and around.

Further Resources

For spinning, consult your local child.

For Sufi dervish, the sounds have been captured on recordings like *Islamic Liturgy: Song and Dance at a Meeting of the Dervishes.* The performance of dervish spinning by the Mevlevi Sufi sect, formerly banned by Turkish law, is now legal and tourists can see weekly ceremonies in Konya, Turkey. There are also educational centers across the United States, where you can learn more about the ritual, view performances, and train to whirl yourself: Check out the Mevlevi Order of America (hayatidede.org), which has branches in California, Washington, Oregon, Hawaii, and Virginia, and the Dervish Retreat Center in upstate New York (whirling-dervish.org).

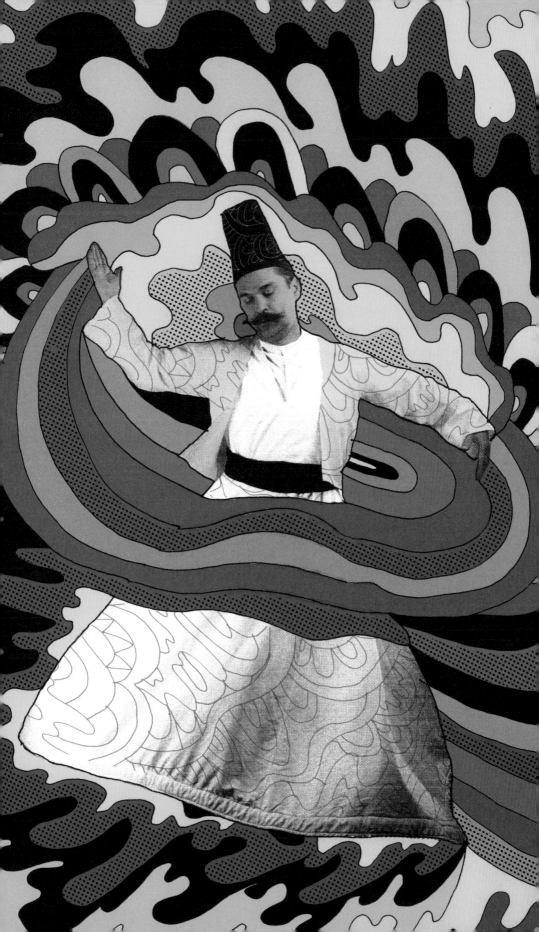

• •

17 Fervent prayer

Prayer conditions by repetition.

I pledge allegiance to the flag of the United States of America, and to the republic for which it stands, one nation, under God, indivisible, with liberty and justice for all.
—THE PLEDGE OF ALLEGIANCE

Our Father, who art in heaven, hallowed be Thy name; Thy kingdom come, Thy will be done on earth as it is in heaven. Give us this day our daily bread and forgive us our trespasses as we forgive those who trespass against us, and lead us not into temptation but deliver us from evil. Amen.
—THE LORD'S PRAYER

I believe in God, the Father almighty, Creator of heaven and earth, and in Jesus Christ, His only son, our Lord, who was conceived by the Holy Spirit and born of the Virgin Mary.
—FROM THE APOSTLES' CREED

Hear, oh Israel, the Lord our God, the Lord is one.
—FROM THE JEWISH SH'MA

Sentient beings are numberless; I vow to save them. Desires are inexhaustible; I vow to extinguish them. The Dharmas are boundless; I vow to master them. The Buddha-truth is unsurpassable; I vow to attain it.
—BUDDHIST BODHISATTVA'S VOWS

May heaven and earth swell our nourishment; the two who are father and mother, all knowing, doing wondrous work. Communicative and wholesome unto all, may heaven and earth bring unto us gain, reward and riches.
—FROM THE HINDU RIG VEDA

Praise be to Allah, Lord of the Worlds, The Beneficent, the Merciful. Owner of the Day of Judgment, Thee alone we worship; Thee alone we ask for help. Show us the straight path, The path of those whom Thou hast favored; Not the path of those who earn Thine anger nor of those who go astray.
—THE KORAN, CHAPTER 1, VERSE 2

The Tao that can be told of is not the Eternal Tao. The names that can be named are not the eternal names. The Way of Heaven is to benefit, not to do harm. The Way of the sage is to act without striving.
—FROM THE TAO TE CHING

He who offends the gods has no one to whom he can pray.
—FROM CONFUCIUS'S ANALECTS

Fervent prayer is glowing, insistent, and passionate.
Fervent prayer does not end; it burns within like fire.
Make up your own prayer; find your own God.
Pray over and over. Pour your prayer from your belly.
Be your prayer.

Prayer conditions by repetition.

Prayer conditions by repetition.

Prayer conditions by repetition.

Prayer conditions by repetition.

Further Resources

The emerging field of neurotheology examines what occurs in the brain during religious experiences. When researcher Andrew Newberg examined brain scans of Franciscan nuns in prayer, he found increased activity in the frontal lobes, which are associated with heightened states of focus (like meditation) and decreased activity in the orientation area of the brain, which is linked to our perception of space and time. Newberg suggests that this creates the feelings of transcendence sometimes associated with a state of fervent prayer. For a further explanation of Newberg's work, see his books *How God Changes Your Brain* and *Principles of Neurotheology*.

18 Long times at sea, in the desert, in the Arctic

Nature challenges and rewards.

At sea the weather is obvious, it is paramount. High and low pressure rule life with pull and tug, rising and falling. The water becomes a seething paradox, one wave to another, one wave becoming another. Where do the waves go? The color of the sky is the color of water. Or is the color of the water the color of the sky?

To sail around the world. To take a boat and leave land and stay only with the water. Our earth is more than three-quarters ocean and sea. Our bodies are water. We need water. We are water.

In the desert there is little water. There is wind. There is sand and heat and brush. Sometimes there is glare and sometimes gloom, but always life. Going to the desert is leaving water behind, abandoning the vegetation or the concrete of our prior abode. The desert is one of the great extremes. The desert is where most of the masters go for their ultimate journey before returning to their communities. The desert is the test. When the sun is high the desert is the clear white light. Altered states of all kinds are certainly a major focus of desert festivals today, like Burning Man. Though some attend to use chemicals, others get high by just being there, dressing up and down, and making all kinds of creative artworks.

The clear white light of the Arctic and Antarctic regions goes on for days and weeks and months. The Arctic is snow and ice. White. No end in sight. Miles and miles of white in the cold. Only the wind and the sky are ever present. There is no year-round life there, save small, wingless insects and the penguin. To live in this environment is to pare down existence to the wind and cold and ice and snow and sky. To be alone. To be. Like the silent Eskimo, sitting, doing nothing in his igloo, waiting for better weather.

Further Resources

W. Gibson's *The Boat,* J. Slocum's *Sailing Alone Around the World,* and E. W. Anderson's article for the *Journal of the Royal Naval Medical Service,* "Abnormal Mental States in Survivors, with Special Reference to Collective Hallucinations" (1942) pretty much cover the experience at sea.

Jesus went to the desert to work it all out, as have many masters before and since. When I asked a friend of Claudio Naranjo what the former Gestalt therapist was doing in Chile, studying with Oscar Ichazo, I was told that "Claudio is in the desert now for eighty days. He gets an egg and an orange every other day." A similar but self-directed isolation experience is recounted in Tom Neale's *An Island to Myself.*

C. Byrd's book *Alone* describes an Arctic experience, as does Christiane Ritter's *A Woman in the Polar Night.* Edmund Carpenter's classic study is titled *Eskimo.*

19 Self-hypnosis
Your trance is getting deeper . . .

Self-hypnosis is an easy and pleasant way to alter consciousness. To induce self-hypnosis an object for the focus of your attention is needed. Anything will do; the best is a candle. Take a candle to a place where you will be comfortable and undisturbed. Light it.

You are going to hypnotize yourself by convincing yourself, through self-suggestion, that you are in a trance. Hypnotic induction also requires the selection of a key word or phrase, for use while you are hypnotizing yourself. Here are some examples:

Deeper

Now

Heavy

Further

I'm relaxed

I'm going deeper

My trance is getting deeper

To begin self-hypnosis, select a comfortable position, either sitting or lying down, and look at the candle. Don't stare at the candle for long periods of time. The purpose of the candle is to provide a centering point so that your consciousness will slip into a trance. As you look at the flame give yourself the following instructions: "I am growing sleepy. My eyelids are getting heavier and heavier. I am sinking away. I can't keep my eyes open." Accompany these instructions with full, deep breathing.

Once your eyes begin to close, you are entering the beginning of the hypnotic trance. Now is the time for your key word. The word is used to deepen your trance. Stay with your key word by repeating it as often as you can.

At this stage it is important to relax. As you repeat your key word, send your consciousness to each part of your body. If you find a tight, tensed area, loosen it. Do this until you are in a completely relaxed state. This relaxation deepens and enriches your trance.

Now begin counting backward, slowly, from ten to one. As you count, imagine yourself traveling downward deeper into your own self. Let your eyelids become heavy. Concentrate on the different parts of your body. Let each part become very heavy and sink, just as you yourself are sinking into a deep, deep trance. Your limbs become heavier and you become heavier. Now lighten the different parts of your body. Let your limbs float up and away. You are floating away. Deeper and deeper, further and further, higher and higher.

To end self-hypnosis simply give yourself the instruction "Now I will end my trance and wake up." You will wake up feeling fine and refreshed.

You can use self-hypnosis to cope with insomnia, increase your powers of concentration, overcome your bad habits, or just take a trip. What is most important in self-hypnosis is attitude. Skepticism, negative expectations, and tension will interfere. If you think that hypnosis will be positive, effective, and helpful, and that you will be able to enter a trance easily, stay in your trance to accomplish your goals, and end your trance without discomfort, then self-hypnosis is absolutely possible.

In the realm of the mind, whatever we think is true, either is true or becomes true.
—JOHN LILLY

Further Resources

The works of Milton Erickson and Bernard Aaronson, in the *American Journal of Clinical Hypnosis,* cover this field very nicely. Charles Tart's book *Altered States of Consciousness* has some interesting papers and some good suggestions for further reading. Two good popular books on this subject include *Self Hypnotism* by Leslie LeCron and *Self-Hypnosis* by Laurance Sparks.

Aaronson's paper "The Hypnotic Induction of the Void," which was presented at the meetings of the American Society of Clinical Hypnosis in San Francisco in 1969, has also been highly praised.

· ·

20 Alterations of breathing

Take a deep breath . . .

Our breath is our life. Air is the first food of the newborn. When we stop breathing, our life ends. Breath nourishes the circulatory system and the brain, the seat of the nervous system. When we alter our breathing, we alter our consciousness and our life.

Throughout our days, our breathing is secondary to our daily concerns for job, family, safety. Breath is in the background. We don't pay attention to our breathing, except in an emergency. People in a burning theater will trample each other because of breathing difficulties. Weights on the chest and diaphragm and swimming under water bring about increased attention to breathing.

To begin conscious and controlled alteration of breathing requires an awareness of the "how" of breathing. Do you inhale through your nose, your mouth, or both? What about exhaling? Pay attention to your breathing for five minutes, and ignore everything but the rhythm and flow of your inhaling and exhaling, the current of your life.

How do you breathe? Is it with your shoulders, chest, ribs, back, or stomach? What combinations do you use? When you take a deep breath, *what* do you take? Where does it go? When you inhale, *what* do you get? When you exhale, what do you lose? What happens in between inhaling and exhaling? Pay attention and find out.

When you breathe too much, too quickly, you can lose consciousness. When you breathe too little, for too long, you can lose consciousness. Either of these alterations of your normal breathing changes the mixture of oxygen that goes to your brain. That mixture is of a delicate balance and to change it subtly or profoundly changes consciousness.

Close your eyes and deeply and fully inhale and exhale five times. Draw the air in through your mouth all the way down, filling your diaphragm, until the breath reaches the pit of your abdomen. When you have brought this air all the way down, pause, and then begin to let the air back up. Make sure that you exhale completely; that all of the air taken in is expired. At the completion of the expiration, pause and then begin the process all over again.

After this experiment, open your eyes and look at your world. Notice the movement, the brightening of colors, the charged atmosphere that surrounds you.

Next, sit in front of a clock or a watch with a sweep second hand or a smartphone with a stopwatch. Hold your breath for as long as you can with your eyes open. Once you know how long that is, do it again, but this time hold your breath longer. Now try the same experiment with your eyes closed. If you are having trouble improving on your time, try watching the sweep of the second hand or the tick of the stopwatch, or setting yourself a specific goal.

Panting, rapid intake and outbreath, and hissing also change consciousness. When you are breathing correctly you will experience your breath "breathing" you. You don't draw air into your body, nor do you push air out of your body; the air flows in and out of its own volition. In between this inhaling and exhaling are natural pauses.

Healthy breathing brings about new consciousness.

The results of these breathing experiments will be an alteration of awareness.

While breathwork originated in practices like yoga and meditation, there are also many contemporary breathing techniques with roots in the 1960s and '70s. For instance, Holotropic Breathwork, developed by Dr. Stan Grof and his wife, Christina, stemmed from their research into consciousness-altering drugs like LSD. Holotropic Breathwork teaches a series of ways of breathing to, as Grof says, "transcend the narrow boundaries of the body and reclaim our full identity." Another Sixties-era breathing technique is Rebirthing Breathwork, developed by Leonard Orr.

The Vaults of Erowid notes: "Changing one's pattern of breathing can influence the mixture of gases entering the bloodstream, triggering physiological effects as well as cognitive changes ranging from mild stimulation to panic. . . . Forms of controlled breath that resemble asphyxiation can have fatal consequences. The 'fainting game' or 'choking game,' sometimes engaged in by young people, is typically done by one person to another.

Though its effects are sometimes described in terms of its psychoactivity, it can also be deadly."

In his book *Heaven and Hell,* Aldous Huxley suggests that by altering breathing, we are increasing the amount of CO_2 in the lungs and blood, which disrupts the function of the "cerebral reducing valve" that moderates the full capacity of our consciousness. Huxley writes, "this, though the shouters, singers, and mutterers do not know it, has been at all times the real purpose and point of magic spells, of mantras, litanies, psalms, and sutras."

Further Resources

Most of the source material and notes listed under Yoga (No. 149) deal with breathing as a way of altering states of consciousness. Also see "Breathing Therapy" by Magda Proskauer in H. Otto and J. Mann's *Ways of Growth.* Stan Grof's Holotropic Breathwork resources can be found on his website (holotropicbreathworkla.com). Kylea Taylor has written two books on Grof's holotropic breathing techniques: the introductory *The Breathwork Experience* and the more advanced *Exploring Holotropic Breathwork. Science Daily* reported that the CART (Capnometry-Assisted Respiratory Training) technique of breathing, developed at Southern Methodist University, has been shown to be helpful in helping patients control panic disorders.

· ·

21 Trance

From hypnosis to electronic dance music, an evolving altered state.

To be dazed, to be detached from your surroundings, to be possessed of your own inner state, is to be in a trance. To be absorbed in your own personal world, forsaking the reality of the world at large, is to be in a trance.

In a trance, there is no functioning, no contact. The usual attachments to our senses, our environment, our bodies, and our feelings are left behind. Only inner consciousness is involved in trance.

To the outside observer those in a trance appear otherworldly, possessed, occupied by something alien or foreign.

In trance, the channels of communication to the brain seem to be disconnected: information cannot get through.
—STEWART WAVELL

Who is it then who enters a trance?

The word "trance" has often been associated with hypnosis, but its meaning in the West has been broadened to include any state of consciousness "other than normal consciousness." Many would agree that the trance state is often achieved in correspondence with trance music and raves, even without the use of drugs. As Oliver Sacks says in *Hallucinations*: "One of the most dramatic effects of music's power is the induction of trance states. . . . Trance—ecstatic singing and dancing, wild movements and cries, perhaps rhythmic rocking, or catatonia-like rigidity or immobility . . . [is a] profoundly altered state."

Further Resources

The book *Trances* by Stewart Wavell, A. Butt, and N. Epton covers some interesting anthropological aspects of trance. *Freedom in Exile* by the Dali Lama of Tibet gives a very complete description of trance states.

22 Myths, tales, and koans

Stories have much to reveal to us.

Myths, tales, and koans represent humankind's most direct attempt to encode his wisdom and make it accessible, communicable, and durable.

Myths usually involve the exploits of a hero or archetypal character who undergoes interactions and transformations at the hands of a real or imaginary environment.

Tales are narrative descriptions of events, often truthful as well as fictitious, usually in the form of a story—that is, a plot with a beginning, middle, and end.

Koan is the Japanese form of the Chinese word *kung-an,* which means, literally, "case," as in a legal case. In the practice of Ch'an and Zen Buddhism, koans refer to stories describing the behavior and the conversations of a Ch'an or Zen master. Here, I use the term "koan" to describe stories relating to the words and activities of various masters in religious groups with a mystical tradition, as well as in groups that have developed methods for altering consciousness. Some of these groups include Ch'an and Zen Buddhism, the Sufis, and the Hasidim.

Myths

Herodotus tells us of the myth of a famous bird, the phoenix, known as a creature that rises from its own ashes:

> This bird comes but seldom into Egypt, once in five hundred years. It is told that the phoenix comes when his father dies. His plumage is partly gold and partly red and he is most like an eagle in shape and in size.

In Chinese mythology, the phoenix is a bird of great beauty, very much like the peacock. There were two types of phoenix, male and female, *feng* and *huang.* When the phoenix chose to visit the court of an emperor, this was a sign of extreme cosmic favor. When *feng* and *huang* are together it is the symbol of everlasting love.

Tales

The Emperor's New Clothes

Many years ago there was an Emperor who was so excessively fond of new clothes that he spent all his money on them. He had a costume for every hour in the day, and instead of saying as one does about any other King or Emperor, "He is in his council chamber," here one always said, "The Emperor is in his dressing-room."

Life was very gay in the great town where he lived; hosts of strangers came to visit it every day, and among them one day two swindlers. They gave themselves out as weavers, and said that they knew how to weave the most beautiful stuffs imaginable. Not only were the colors and patterns unusually fine, but the clothes that were made of the stuffs had the peculiar quality of becoming invisible to every person who was not fit for the office he held, or if he was impossibly dull.

"Those must be splendid clothes," thought the Emperor. "By wearing them I should be able to discover which men in my kingdom are unfitted for their posts. I shall distinguish the wise men from the fools. Yes, I certainly must order some of that stuff to be woven for me."

He paid the two swindlers a lot of money in advance, so that they might begin their work at once.

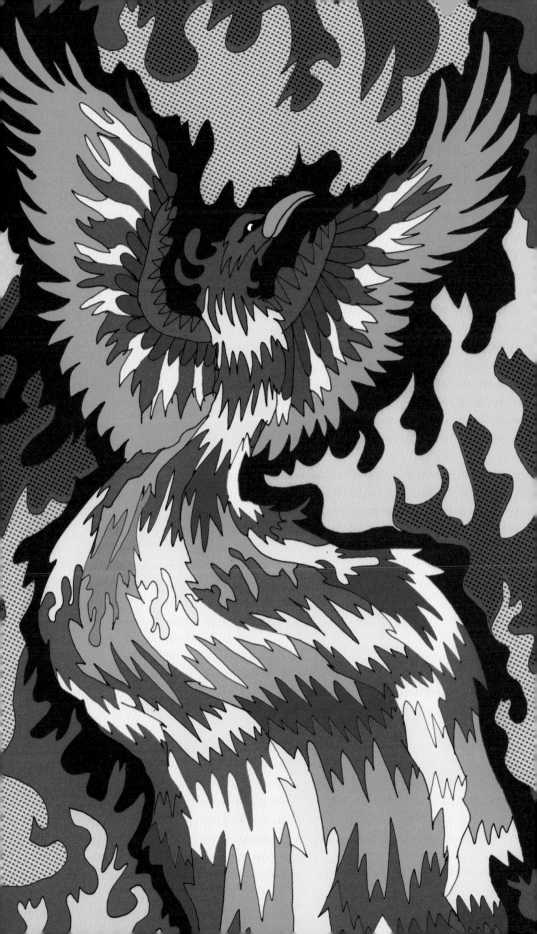

They did put up two looms and pretended to weave, but they had nothing whatever upon their shuttles. At the outset they asked for a quantity of the finest silk and the purest gold thread, all of which they put into their own bags while they worked away at the empty looms far into the night. . . .

"I will send my faithful old minister to the weavers," thought the Emperor. "He will be best able to see how the stuff looks, for he is a clever man and no one fulfills his duties better than he does!"

So the good old minister went into the room where the two swindlers sat working at the empty loom.

"Heaven preserve us!" thought the old minister, opening his eyes very wide. "Why, I can't see a thing!" But he took care not to say so.

Both the swindlers begged him to be good enough to step a little nearer, and asked if he did not think it a good pattern and beautiful coloring. . . .

"Good heavens!" thought he, "is it possible that I am a fool? I have never thought so, and nobody must know it. Am I not fit for my post? It will never do to say that I cannot see the stuffs."

"Well, sir, you don't say anything about the stuff," said the one who was pretending to weave.

"Oh, it is beautiful! Quite charming!" said the minister looking through his spectacles; "This pattern and these colors! I will certainly tell the Emperor that the stuff pleases me very much."

"We are delighted to hear you say so," said the swindlers, and then they named all the colors and described the peculiar pattern. The old minister paid great attention to what they said, so as to be able to repeat it when he got home to the Emperor.

Then the swindlers went on to demand more money, more silk, and more gold, to be able to proceed with the weaving; but they put it all into their own pockets—not a single strand was ever put onto the loom, but they went on as before weaving at the empty loom. . . .

Now the Emperor thought he would like to see it while it was still on the loom. So, accompanied by a number of selected courtiers, among whom were the faithful officials who had already seen the imaginary stuff, he went to visit the craft impostors, who were working away as hard as ever they could at the empty loom.

"It is magnificent!" said the honest officials. "Only see, your Majesty, what a design! What colors!" And they pointed to the empty loom, for they thought no doubt the others could see the stuff.

"What!" thought the Emperor; "I see nothing at all! This is terrible! Am I a fool? Am I not fit to be Emperor? Why, nothing worse could happen to me!"

"Oh, it is beautiful!" said the Emperor. "It has my highest approval!" and he nodded his satisfaction as he gazed at the empty loom. Nothing could induce him to say that he could not see anything. . . .

The Emperor gave each of the rogues an order of knighthood to be worn in their buttonholes and the title of "Gentlemen weavers."

The swindlers sat up the whole night, before the day on which a procession was to take place, burning sixteen candles so that people might see how anxious they were to get the Emperor's new clothes ready. . . . At last they said: "Now the Emperor's new clothes are ready!"

The Emperor, with his grandest courtiers, went to them himself, and both swindlers raised one arm in the air, as if they were holding something, and said: "See, these are the trousers, this is the coat, here is the mantle!" and so on. "It is as light as a spider's web. One might think one had nothing on, but that is the very beauty of it! . . .

"Will your imperial majesty be graciously pleased to take off your clothes," said the imposters, "so that we may put on the new ones, along here before the great mirror."

The Emperor took off all his clothes, and the impostors pretended to give him one article of dress after the other, of the new ones which they had pretended to make. . . .

"Well, I am quite ready," said the Emperor. "Don't the clothes fit well?" and then he turned round again in front of the mirror, so that he should seem to be looking at his grand things. . . .

Then the Emperor walked along in the procession under the gorgeous canopy, and everybody in the streets and at the windows exclaimed, "How beautiful the Emperor's new clothes are! What a splendid train! And they fit to perfection!" Nobody would let it appear that he could see nothing, for then he would not be fit for his post, or else he was a fool.

None of the Emperor's clothes had been so successful before.

"But he has got nothing on," said a little child.

"Oh, listen to the innocent," said its father; and one person whispered to the other what the child had said. "He has nothing on; a child says he has nothing on!"

"But he has nothing on!" at last cried all the people.

The Emperor writhed, for he knew it was true, but he thought "the procession must go on now," so held himself stiffer than ever, and the chamberlains held up the invisible train.

—FROM ANDERSEN'S FAIRY TALES, TRANS. E. LUCAS AND H.B. PAULL

Koans

A monk once asked Chao Chou: "Does a dog have Buddha nature?" [In Buddhism, all sentient beings are possessed of the Buddha nature.] Chao Chou replied: "Wu!" [Wu is Chinese for "no."]

Rabbi Leib, son of Sarah, the hidden zaddik [leader of the Hasidic community] who wandered over the Earth, following the course of rivers in order to redeem the souls of the living and the dead, said this:

"I did not go to the maggid [preacher] in order to hear Torah from him, but to see how he unlaces his felt shoes and laces them up again."

—FROM BUBER, TALES OF HASIDIM, EARLY MASTERS

One evening a Sufi dervish was passing when he heard a voice cry out from deep in a well. He looked down into the well and called out: "What is wrong?"

A voice yelled back in reply: "It is me, the grammarian. I did not know my way and in error fell into this well. And now I'm stuck."

The Sufi replied: "Do not worry, dear man. I will go immediately and bring a rope and a ladder."

As the Sufi started to leave, a voice cried up to him: "Oh, sir. Before you go, please correct your grammar. What you said before was improper in its construction."

To this the Sufi responded: "If this grammar is so essential to your well-being, then please stay right there, and I will go and learn to speak correctly."

So saying, the Sufi left and continued on his way.

—DERIVED FROM RUMI AND SHAH

Hsueh Feng, Wen Sui, and Yen Tou were sitting together. Wen
Sui pointed to a bowlful of water and said: "The moon appears in
the clear water."

Hsueh Feng said: "The moon does not appear in the clear water."

Yen Tou kicked over the bowl of water.

—FROM *THE LIGHTHOUSE IN THE OCEAN OF CH'AN*

Myths and tales provide the seeds of time-wrought expanded awareness for
all of us in our multitude of cultural origins and experiences. In doing so,
they provide lessons from the past that teach us how to live more fully in
the present. Koans, in particular, through their innovative use of language,
challenge us to consider new ways of being, alternative realities.

Further Resources

For myths, see Robert Graves's *The Greek Myths;* Joseph Campbell's
four-volume *The Masks of God,* and his *The Hero with a Thousand Faces;*
Bulfinch's Mythology; and J. Frazer's *The Golden Bough.*

For tales, look back on the collections of the Brothers Grimm; H. C.
Andersen; Borges's *The Book of Imaginary Beings;* and T. H. White's *The
Bestiary.*

Included under Koans are not only stories of the Ch'an and Zen masters, but also those of Sufism and Hasidism.

For Ch'an and Zen koans: *Zen Dust,* by I. Miura and R. Sasaki (also avail-
able in an abbreviated version under the title *The Zen (Koan); Zen and Zen
Classics* (Volume Four: *Mumonkan*) by R. H. Blyth; *Original Teachings of
Ch'an Buddhism* by Chang Chung-Yuan; *Zen Flesh, Zen Bones* by Reps;
The Blue Cliff Records by R. D. M. Shaw; *The Embossed Tea Kettle* by
Hakuin Zenji; *The Iron Flute* by Senzaki and McCandless; *The Practice of
Zen* by Chang Chen Chi; *The Golden Age of Zen* by J. C. H. Wu; *Tai Hsu* by
Chou Hsiang Kuang; *Dhyana Buddhism in China* by the same author; John
Blofeld's *The Zen Teaching of Huang Po* and *The Zen Teaching of Hui Hai;*
and *The Lighthouse in the Ocean of Ch'an* by C. M. Chen. The Sufi Tales:
The Recountings of Idries Shah, *The Sufis; The Way of the Sufi; Tales of the
Dervishes; Wisdom of the Idiots; The Exploits of the Incomparable Mulla
Nasrudin* and *The Pleasantries of the Incredible Mulla Nasrudin;* also A. J.
Arberry's *Sufism.*

Martin Buber collected many stories of the Hasidim in his two-volume
Tales of the Hasidim, Early Masters and *Later Masters.*

. . . .

23 Rituals

To transcend, you must first master the ceremony.

When men did everything to please their gods, things had to be done the correct way each and every time. This was especially true of ceremonies. Rites of passage, rites of initiation, appeals for an end to a state of ill health—all of these demanded a form for communicating with the gods. Ritual provided this form and today still provides access to other, nonordinary states of reality. The exactness of any ritual procedure endows the actions with a very unique spirit. This spirit can be felt in even the most ordinary of circumstances.

A familiar example of a ritual is the school graduation ceremony. There are speeches, costumes, and music. There are the elders bestowing power on the new initiates; there are the set and prescribed ways of behaving. Outbursts and walkouts by students might be overlooked during any other time or at any other function of the school year, but the special ritualistic atmosphere of the graduation ceremonies make such departures from expected behavior much more outrageous.

As an experiment, designate a particular time to perform a ritual each week. Stay with this schedule for at least a month. The repetition over that long a period of time will enable the ritual to take on a spirit that will at once surprise, inform, and exhilarate you.

Ingredients might include things such as prayers, incantations, and movements. Other, more material ritual ingredients might include musical instruments, various liquids (preferably of many colors), fabrics, plants and objets d'art. Be imaginative and combine these things into an ordered, structured, and repeatable ceremony. This ceremony will be your ritual.

Further Resources

Most social groups, societies, and tribes have special rituals. The American Indians have some really beautiful ones outlined and described in Frank Waters's books *Book of the Hopi* and *Masked Gods*. Haile, Oakes, and Wyman provide a detailed description of one Navajo ceremony in *Beautyway*. Frazer's *The Golden Bough* provides a good starting point for introductory material.

24 Chanting and mantras

Fill your body with the power of your voice.

C hanting is one of the most effective ways to turn on without drugs. It may take a little more time than some of the other techniques, but it always gets good results.

Chanting is a particular way of making sound with the human voice involving repetition of sound and tone. In some chants each syllable is held for an entire breath; in others a breath is taken only when needed. No matter which way you chant, the main idea is to develop your breathing through your chanting. By changing your normal breathing through chanting you will be increasing the oxygen level of the blood reaching your brain and, thereby, alter your consciousness.

A great chant for Westerners is the chanting of your own name. In his workshops on chanting, Bernard Aaronson instructed the group members to chant their own names: *BER—NARD—AAR—ON—SON*.

Hindus, Buddhists, and others chant holy syllables known as mantrum. A very holy mantra, sometimes called the sound of God, is: *OM*.

Mantras are taken to be the sound of the universe and are chanted for the vibrational quality that they stimulate in the chanter. Chanters and singers on the streets of many American cities made the Hare Krishna chant popular. The chant: *HARE KRISHNA, HARE KRISHNA, KRISHNA, KRISHNA, HARE; HARE RAMA, HARE RAMA, RAMA RAMA, HARE HARE*.

There are also Western mantras. President John F. Kennedy used to chant: *GO! GO! GO! GO! GO! GO! GO! GO!*

There is a chant used to expel evil that comes from the Gnostic tradition. The chant removes one letter with each new intonation. The "s" at the end of each word is always hissed:

ABROXSIS

BROXSIS

ROXSIS

OXSIS

XSIS

SIS

IS

S

LIVE VERY RICHLY YOU HAPPY ONE is based on the chakras of Tantric Yoga. The seven chakras are energy centers that are located along the spine. Six of the seven centers have a mantra. The seventh and highest chakra, the thousand-petaled lotus at the crown of the head, has a silent mantra. The sound of each mantra in this chant is represented by the first letter of each word in the sentence: LIVE VERY RICHLY YOU HAPPY ONE.

This chant takes about thirty minutes. Begin by sitting on the floor in a comfortable position. Make sure that your spine and neck are straight and erect. Start chanting the first mantra: **LUM.**

Chant **LUM** for five minutes. As you chant, summon the power from the base of your spine and start it on a journey upward. Remember to take deep breaths, and as you chant let the sound continue until you have let out all of your breath. As you chant you will experience the vibratory power of your voice increasing. Fill your body with your chanting.

Now, after chanting *LUM* for five minutes, go on to the next mantra: **VUM.**

Continue chanting this mantra for five minutes. This procedure is repeated for each mantra:

LUM

VUM

RUM

YUM

HUM

OM

After you chant *OM*, start five minutes of silent contemplation. The sound vibrations from the previous chanting will fill the spaces around you with energy. Work to move this energy up your spine through your neck and finally into your head. Your breathing, your vibrations, and your energy will turn you on.

Further Resources

Numerous books on chanting are available. See resources for Yoga (No. 149), Buddhism (No. 157), Tibetan Buddhism (No. 152) and Sufism (No. 165).

To listen to chants, consult the following albums and songs that are available on the *Book of Highs* Spotify playlist: *The Music of Tibet* (from the Gyuto Multiphonic Choir, recorded by Huston Smith); the UNESCO Collection's *Tibetan Ritual* with invocations performed by Buddhist monks; "Jilala" (North African Sufi chanting ceremony); *Music from the Morning of the World* (The Balinese Gamelan); "Hare Krishna (Maha Mantra)" by the Indian classical singer Jagit Singh; and "Rakhay Rakhanhaar," by Ram Dass.

25 Mudra

Hand positions for greater peace.

Mudras are symbols, hand positions created by placing the hands and fingers in certain prescribed ways that represent a variety of metaphysical states or conditions. They were developed as expressions for Hindu and Buddhist ceremonies and are often used in religious iconography.

Mudra are used by priests at religious ceremonies. Under these circumstances mudra have a highly specialized and ritualistic function, but they can be isolated from their religious setting and used for personal expression and creativity. The use of mudra requires a high degree of discipline. They can bring about unique aesthetic experiences.

The religious uses of mudra provide some three hundred separate but often highly repetitious positions for the hands and fingers. There are fourteen basic positions which, when varied, yield about forty differing forms of mudra.

Sit in a chair or cross-legged on the floor with your back straight in a quiet room. Using the illustration provided here, try out some of the mudra positions. Start with the simple, open-handed positions and gradually work your way to the more complex configurations. You will be able to experience the different ways in which mudra affect your consciousness as you let the energy generated by a specific hand position flow through your entire body.

When your right hand is open and raised up by your shoulder and your left hand is placed palm up in front of your stomach, you will feel openness and receptivity. By holding this position for extended periods you will enhance peacefulness and tranquility. Other mudra engender different consciousness experiences. In the beginning use a mirror to ensure that your position is correct. Hold the position for sixty seconds or so and slowly move to the next.

Further Resources

E. Dale Saunders's *Mudra* is the classic study. It is detailed and easy to read and includes copious references to supplementary material for further study. Many of the books listed under the resources for Yoga (No. 149), Tibetan Buddhism (No. 152), and Buddhism (No. 157.) also include material on mudra and their use.

26 Problem solving

Finding new ways of being.

None of us looks forward to problems. They try us, tax our faculties, and often frustrate us and make us uncomfortable. They make life difficult.

They also make life vital, arresting, engaging, and interesting. They allow us to tap into our potential. They make demands on us. Problems often require that we bring a new and unaccustomed viewpoint to a situation. It is in the experience of both the positive *and* the negative aspects of problems that we can find ways to change thought and action, the ways in which we experience the world and the ways we are. Problems provide us with the opportunity to explore fresh new ways of being.

The most important thing to remember when using problem solving as a method for altering your consciousness is to remain open to the opportunity to experience and sense what you have not previously been aware of.

Another key to problem solving as a way to get high is persistence. By sticking with a problem, reviewing past procedures, and evaluating current status, you can make the obvious and the overlooked become clear. This often brings out the problem's solution and, along with the solution, the feeling of insight and closure: "a-ha!"

A good example of problem solving is attempting to discover what it is about your relationship with someone that makes you dislike each other. It might be something in their personality that you dislike, whereas further reflection and insight could make it clear that what you see in them that is distasteful is something you find in yourself that you try to hide. Or it might be that when you hear the other person speak you don't like what they say. If you recognize this as a problem, you can enable yourself to listen more openly and perhaps hear what the other is really saying. This in turn may lead to discoveries about how you talk and what you say. These experiences can lead to new insights about other people and about you.

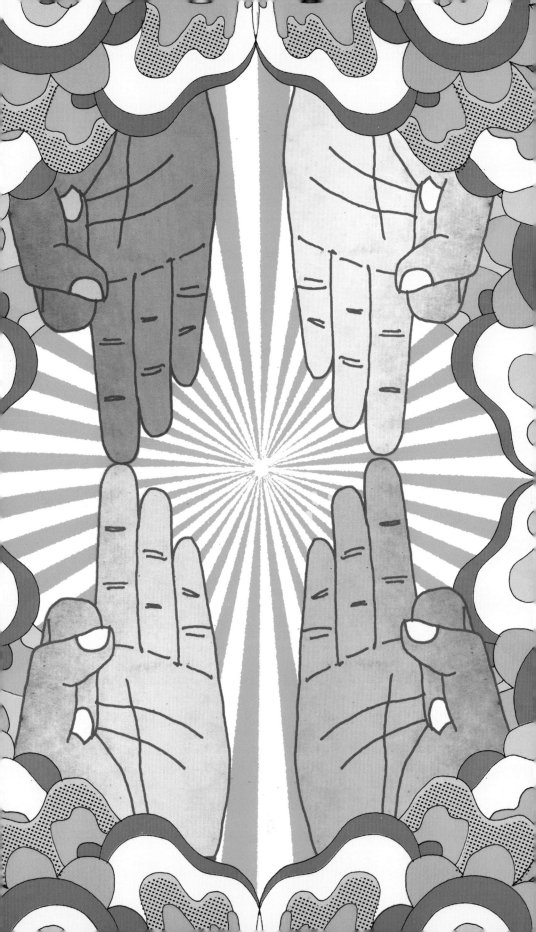

....

27 Extra-sensory perception

Transcend the limits of your senses.

Extra-sensory perception (ESP) is the ability to perceive the environment without, or over and above, the limits of the senses. Most people experience ESP as a strange feeling, often like a hunch or intuition. Along with this feeling comes a knowledge, for example, that the next card to be upturned from a deck will be the ace of hearts. That particular type of experience is known as precognition and is one of the easiest of the ESP phenomena to test in a laboratory. These types of tests were performed in the 1920s by J. B. and Louisa Rhine and their associates at Duke University. They made up a new deck of cards with five suits, established the statistical probability of guessing which suit would appear at any given time, and then set about testing both normal people and those who claimed to have precognitive abilities.

Testing has continued today and now includes experiments that test for psychokinesis (the ability to move material with mental power), out-of-body travel, ESP dream influence, and the predicting of events.

A more recent take on the importance of ESP comes from the author Daniel Pinchbeck, who refers to the phenomenon by its other name, psi: "Psi could be exponentially more powerful as a transformative force than electricity, if we can figure out how to use it." Here Pinchbeck is taking the lead from psychologist Lawrence LeShan, who noted: "We must be open to facing the possibility that we will find things so new and startling that they change our preconceptions about ourselves and the universe we live in. So far, we have not had that courage. Perhaps now with species extinction looming before us we will find that courage."

You can practice ESP yourself and try to develop your own paranormal powers. Devise some of your own experiments, but remember to start slowly. Don't try to move the living-room couch with your mind power as an opener. First try card guessing. With five different cards you should be able to guess right about one out of five cards, and so on. If you seem to do much better than average, try communicating with your friends and relatives by thought power alone and observe the results. If you have real ESP abilities, contact one of the groups referred to in Further Resources and they will submit your talents to rigid scientific testing.

Further Resources

The Parapsychology Foundation's website (parapsychology.org) offers plenty of useful information, as does the American Society for Psychical Research (aspr.com). Dr. Stanley Krippner, who conducted research on ESP as well as biofeedback and other subjects as the director of the Menninger Dream Laboratory at Maimonides Medical Center in Brooklyn, still writes about the subject on his website (stanleykrippner.weebly.com). Some of the results of ESP work in Eastern European countries are chronicled in Ostrander and Schroeder's *Psychic Discoveries Behind the Iron Curtain.* Lawrence LeShan's *A New Science of the Paranormal* is still an excellent source of rational discourse about the irrational. Daniel Pinchbeck's description of the role of psi in the future is covered in *How Soon Is Now: From Personal Initiation to Global Transformation.* The details of the most extensive, government-backed ESP research in the United States are the basis of the book *Phenomena* by Annie Jacobsen.

28 Culturally based visual illusions

How your culture controls what you see.

Our brains and our eyes constantly compensate for the raw material we perceive in our environment. Our culture and geographic location adds to the distortions we perceive.

We see clearly into the distance when we look out on a landscape, but do not when looking down, at objects a shorter distance away, from a very high building or structure. People who live in the forest do not perceive distance at all, since there are only small clear areas in that environment.

Take the "carpentered world" hypothesis, which emerged in the 1960s, and is still being researched today. Cultures that emphasize straight lines and right angles in their architecture experience certain "straight line" illusions (like the Müller-Lyer effect), whereas cultures like the Zulu, who live in a "round" world—with round buildings and round doors and round everyday objects—do not perceive straight lines and their attendant illusions.

Our location in the universe also creates attendant illusions. The Earth revolves in a solar orbit, yet we see the sun "rise" in the morning and "set" in the evening; and man has yet to arrive at a satisfactory explanation of why the moon looks bigger when it rises than it does when it reaches mid-sky.

It might be difficult to imagine in today's screen-focused society, but in the past, only Westerners knew how to watch a screen full of images by focusing directly *in front* of the screen, rather than looking *at* the screen. People not trained this way saw only a portion of what occurs on the screen at any given time. Usually they were not able to integrate what they saw into any meaningful, organized whole. Marshall McLuhan, in *The Guttenberg Galaxy,* tells the story of the educational film about drainage of stagnant pools of water shown to African villagers. When asked what they saw, those viewing the film unanimously said they saw "the chicken." When the film was reviewed, frame by frame, there was a fleeting image of a chicken running across the scene for about two seconds. The ways in which consciousness is focused and images are formed are truly culturally determined.

Further Resources

R. L. Gregory's two books *Eye and Brain* and *The Intelligent Eye* provide good background material and suggestions for follow-up and further research. Adam Alter's *Drunk Tank Pink: And Other Unexpected Forces That Shape How We Think, Feel, and Behave* describes the differences in cultural responses to the Müller-Lyer illusion. *Popular Science* ran an excerpt from the chapter "Are These Lines the Same Height? Your Answer Depends on Where You're From" on March 20, 2013.

• •

29 Auditory illusions

If seeing is not believing, neither is hearing.

Our senses can be manipulated with and without our knowledge. Perhaps the most astounding examples of auditory illusions come from Richard Warren of the University of Wisconsin. In conjunction with Richard Gregory of Great Britain, a tape that mechanically repeated a word over and over was devised. After listening to the word, which was different for each subject, each heard a word *other than* the word being played. They heard the new word emphatically, and in most cases were sure that it was part of the tape. Actually the new word was supplied by the brain. Bored with hearing the same word over and over, it created its own diversion.

Another Warren experiment replaced part of a word in a sentence with a cough, and then with a tone. Warren then played the tape to subjects and asked them which part of which word had been obscured. The sentence was:

"The state governors met with their respective legi(s)latures convening in the city capital."

The "s" was replaced first by the cough, and then by the tone. None of the subjects could hear which letter had been obliterated. Some even insisted that there had been no alteration.

More recently, Diana Deutsch of the University of California, San Diego, has studied auditory illusions of speech and music. Her various websites provide powerful examples of many of these auditory illusions—such as her findings and demonstrations of the way in which music and words are deeply intertwined.

Try to create your own auditory illusions. Make up a sentence that you can recite to friends, in which a letter or word is added to or subtracted from a meaningful part of the sentence, much the same way as Warren did on his tape at the University of Wisconsin. See if your friends can hear the difference; ask them what they heard. Another experiment can be to reverse the order of two words in a sentence: "I'm going to dinner eat." See if your friends notice.

Further Resources

Nigel Calder discusses auditory hallucinations in his book *The Mind of Man*. Deutsch's work can be found on her website (deutsch.ucsd.edu) and on *The Book of Highs* YouTube playlist.

• •

30 Afterimages

When the flash of a camera creates a lingering light show.

Afterimages are the visual sensations that we take from a subject of our sight after we leave it and look elsewhere. Perhaps the most familiar of all the afterimages is the one that occurs when a camera flash is used. After the flash goes off, a colored image covers part or all of the visual field of those who were looking at the flash. This image usually persists for several seconds and often changes color.

Other afterimages having to do with bright light come from staring or prolonged observation. Even with a low-watt lightbulb, an afterimage can be created by allowing the light from the bulb to fill the visual field for a brief period of time. An interesting effect occurs when you do this, but with only one eye, keeping the other closed. After looking away, the afterimage will occur only in the open eye, whereas the eye kept closed will perceive monocularly, with normal vision. The mixture of normal vision and vision obscured by a colored afterimage is most dramatic.

There is a sect in India that spends all day looking at the sun as it moves across the sky. Most of the adherents of this sect eventually go blind. Though staring at the sun will produce afterimages, one does not recommend its practice.

Some people experience a different afterimage: the blur. This is much like the effect achieved when one moves a camera while taking a picture. The easiest way to produce these afterimages is to rapidly turn the head left, right, left, and so on.

· ·

31 Repetition
Over and over and over and over and . . .

R epetition is one of the most powerful means of altering consciousness without drugs. It is part of many of the methods outlined in this book. Repetition is essential for all chanting, prolonged observation, most prayer, most hypnotic inductions, a variety of body movements, and even brain-wave feedback.

What makes repetition so effective is that whatever image, sound, or exposure is repeated is then perceived by the observer in a new light. One is enabled to see, hear, taste, smell, feel, or otherwise experience whatever is repeated in new ways. This often leads to an alteration of consciousness.

The other aspect of repetition that makes it powerful is its "overload-ing" quality. It is often when things become too much for us and for our perceptual and experiential systems that we are finally ready to change. Repetition can help bring about those changes. Eat a bowl of berries, notic-ing the differences in them and you. Listen to a word, or a phrase, over and over and over and over and . . .

32 Psychological exercises

Tease your brain.

P sychological exercises are also known as brainteasers or brain twisters. A. R. Orage, who studied with George Gurdjieff and Pytor Ouspensky, provides some good exercises with which one can start. These are to be done subvocally in the head.

Recite Lincoln's Gettysburg Address while counting backward by threes; at the same time, say "Peter Piper picked a peck of pickled peppers," repeatedly.

Make the above exercise more difficult by interspersing the backward number-counting in between every fourth backward-recited word of the Lincoln speech. But do remember to keep repeating "Peter Piper," etc. All of this is to be done subvocally, of course.

Orage also suggests compiling lists of things associated with different parts of the earth, different letters of the alphabet, and so on.

At the same time that you are reading a book, subvocally say "hello" to every inhalation and "goodbye" to every exhalation. Be careful to maintain the integrity of both tasks at once.

Let all of the letters in the alphabet be represented by a number, e.g., a = 1, b = 2, c = 3, x = 24, y = 25, z = 26; and then say something familiar like: "I do." . . . 9, 4, 15. Now try some more difficult sentences.

It's also lots of fun to invent your own psychological exercises.

33 Mathematics

The greatest discoveries require intellectual de-conditioning.

Mathematics is far more interesting than its symbolic language. It is a set of penetrating and arresting ideas. The art of mathematics can be used as a technique for altering states of consciousness. This fact has not been hitherto observed, although mathematical discoverers have gained their primary intuitions of new findings through states of consciousness altered in this manner. The business of discovery is to venture from the familiar into the unfamiliar and relate the latter to the former by means of already known experience, conceptual or sensory. (To discover is at least 1,000 times more difficult than to explain after discovery. The greatest discoveries are not essentially complicated, but they are always unfamiliar, and require intellectual de-conditioning to learn.)
—CHARLES MUSÈS IN "ALTERING STATES OF CONSCIOUSNESS BY MATHEMATICS, WITH APPLICATIONS TO EDUCATION," IN *JOURNAL FOR THE STUDY OF CONSCIOUSNESS*, 3, P. 43.

What is most important when pursuing mathematics as a means of turning on is to proceed into the unfamiliar. It is only in this realm that one will encounter the stimuli and imaginary experience necessary for changing concepts of existence. Though problem solving can be used to turn on (see No. 26), in mathematics it is the voyage into the unknown and the use of mathematics to map the areas investigated and revealed that best contribute to states of altered consciousness.

Stack Exchange's *History of Science and Mathematics* has a section devoted to "Claims of mathematical breakthroughs while in an altered state of consciousness?" There the mathematical discoveries of Poincare, Erdos, and others are examined and their connections to altered states are explained.

Further Resources

The *Journal for the Study of Consciousness* regularly publishes articles by Charles Musès and others about the use of mathematics to alter consciousness. Additional material can be found in *Consciousness and Reality: The Human Pivot Point*, edited by Musès and Arthur M. Young. Stack Exchange: http://hsm.stackexchange.com/questions/3781/claims-of-mathematical-breakthroughs-while-in-an-altered-state-of-consciousness/3785.

• •

34 Continuous singing

Say aaahhh . . . and don't stop.

This technique has been pioneered by La Monte Young and Marian Zazeela, who practice it assiduously. Frequently they travel to India to receive instruction from their singing teacher. You can use their techniques without their extreme dedication. (Other aspects of the work of Young and Zazeela are covered in No. 222.)

Basically, continuous singing is singing a very exacting series of notes and tones in continuous alternating frequencies. It enables you to turn on, much in the same way that chanting does, by altering your breathing and by the ever-present vibrations of the singing itself.

To begin continuous singing, open your mouth as if you were in the doctor's and he wanted to look at the back of your throat. The doctor might ask you to say: "aaahhh." You begin singing by not only saying "aaahhh," loudly and with force, but then turning that "aaahhh" into as melodious and continuous a song as you are capable of. Don't worry about the aesthetics of your sound in the beginning, just work on the continuity of the singing.

Keep singing!!

Try variations on the tone and quality of your "aaahhh," bringing it up and down the register to the best of your ability. It will take at least twenty minutes of this singing for you to turn on. If you really want to think about the potential of this technique, consider the fact that Young and Zazeela try to sing for at least six or more hours each day.

Further Resources

The teacher of Young and Zazeela, Pandit Pran Nath, has an album of his singing titled *Earth Grove.* To listen to a portion of Young's album *Dream House 78' 17"* visit *The Book of Highs* YouTube playlist.

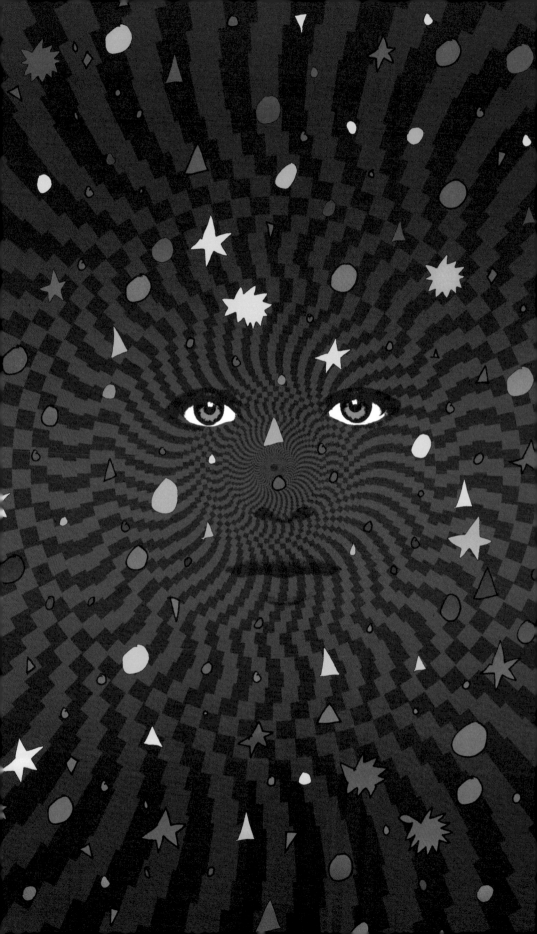

35 Manual phosphene stimulation

May all your eyelid movies be spectaculars.

Phosphenes are the "stars" we see before our eyes. We can see them whenever we want by simply rubbing our closed eyes. Phosphenes are subjective images that are not generated by external visual stimuli. They are produced by the structure of the eye and by the brain.

You don't have to be in the dark to see phosphenes. All you have to do is close your eyes. Spectacular phosphenes can be seen by simply turning your face toward the shower nozzle. The force of the water beating down on the eyelids stimulates a fantastic full-color "light show."

Phosphene stimulation can be put to work anytime, anywhere you can close your eyes. Make sure that your hands are clean. With eyes closed, press your fingertips lightly on your eyeballs near the inside corner of your eyes. Maintaining a steady gentle pressure and motion, rub for about five seconds. You will begin to see "stars." Light pressure creates circular forms like mandalas. More pressure will create more intricate patterns, like spider webs.

May all your eyelid movies be spectaculars.

Further Resources

Gerald Oster's article "Phosphenes," in the February 1970 (Volume 222, Number 2) issue of *Scientific American* gives a complete review of the field, with references for further reading.

36 Zen power yell

Start the day ferociously.

The Zen power yell is a fast way to get in touch with your own personal power and energy.

Begin the Zen power yell from a Japanese sitting position: Sit on your knees with your buttocks perched on the heels of your feet. Keep your arms at your sides.

Begin to breathe fully and deeply. Take a deep breath and then exhale. After letting out your breath, say: "one." Then take another breath, exhale, and say: "two." Repeat through the number five. After saying "five," as you begin to take the next breath, bring your hands up, fists clenched, and cross your arms over your chest. Your left fist should be touching your right shoulder and your right fist should be touching your left shoulder.

Continue your breathing-counting cycle to "eight." After saying "eight," take a deep breath, and suddenly: BOUND UPWARD WITH ALL OF YOUR MIGHT, ROARING LIKE A LION!

Throw your arms out forcefully. In that moment you *are* powerful and ferocious.

The Zen power yell is a great way to greet the world in the morning!

· ·

37 Poetry

The most turned-on language is poetry.

Read poetry aloud.

The beginning of autumn;

The sea and fields,
All one same green.
—BASHO

If you have form'd a Circle to go into,
Go into it yourself & see how you would do.
—WILLIAM BLAKE

Think you, 'mid all this mighty sum
Of things for ever speaking,
That nothing of itself will come,
But we must still be seeking?
—WILLIAM WORDSWORTH

WHO is
Nothing. But all of it's
Everything!
Who is nothing Hear that!
Meaning:
The stars sing
Because it's always all right!
So far you've
Not been near except when
You didn't know. Night's day
Was everywhere. No one is
Ever separated from every other
For then the world would die.
And the world does not die!
O Glory, Glory of the Light!
We live one life. Message ends
—KENNETH PATCHEN

This snowy morning
That black crow
I hate so much . . .
But he's beautiful
—BASHO

· ·

38 Voluntary silence

Be quiet!

You take your language sounds for granted. The easiest way to find out how deeply you are dependent on words is to go without speaking for more than twelve hours. An easy way to turn on is to be silent for two days.

This means: no talking, no moaning, no squeaking, no sounds at all.

"[Buckminster Fuller] spent two years silent after illusory language got him in trouble, and he returned to human communication with a redesigned instrument," writes Stewart Brand in the *Whole Earth Catalog*.

You may return to communication with your own redesigned instrument but you must really be silent.

You might decide never to speak again. Indian spiritual leader Meher Baba started a silence in 1925 that continued until he died in 1969. He often referred to the fact that all the other avatars came with a verbal message that man always ignored. Meher Baba was silent to avoid this pitfall. A 2011 World Health Organization report called noise pollution a "modern plague," stating that "there is overwhelming evidence that exposure to environmental noise has adverse effects on the health of the population."

People who experience silence for long periods might also hear extraordinary sounds.

Further Resources

John Cage's book *Silence*. John Francis, a musician, an activist, and a National Geographic Fellow, was silent for nearly two decades. For the full story of his experience, consult his memoir, *Planetwalker: 22 Years of Walking. 17 Years of Silence,* or his profile in *The Atlantic* ("The Art of Listening: Secrets from 17 Years of Silence," April 26, 2011). Also worth noting: friendsofsilence.net.

· ·

39 Loving

Love someone, or something, but love.
—R. H. BLYTH

Who better to ask about the nature of loving than my wife of more than thirty-five years, Sylvia Rosenfeld? She is a renowned couples and sex therapist in private practice in New York City. Sylvia also supervises and trains psychotherapists.

Sylvia distinguishes between two different kinds of love: the head-over-heels "falling in love," and the more long-lasting attachment love. As for the former, limerence and infatuation are definitely altered states of consciousness. When we fall in love, we are stimulated and feel magically energized. Our sexual desires are heightened and elevated. Our defenses are lowered. This natural high is a result of elevated levels of dopamine and norepinephrine. These chemicals are partner-activated, so we obsessively and passionately seek to be near our loved one or fantasize about them, in order to get the big neurochemical hit. And, for at least several weeks, months, or even more, those hits keep on coming. Couples in monogamous relationships need to create novelty and freshness in order to sustain or re-create their relationships. Couples in polyamorous, open relationships, in addition to being in primary, long-term loving relationships, can find the novelty of infatuation love with others; this is called "new relationship energy."

Attachment love, dare we call it "vintage love," is also often referred to as the quiet love, especially compared to the excitement generated in infatuation loving. This longer-term contact form of loving creates a different high. We feel calm, peaceful, confident, and secure. We feel a sense of oneness, closeness, and connection. The high in this more mature love is produced primarily by the hormones oxytocin and vasopressin; these are often called the cuddle chemicals.

As the late R. H. Blyth, the great writer on Zen, haiku poetry, and Asian culture, observed, how important it is to love: "Love someone, or something, but love."

Further Resources

Some of the best research on love and its chemical constituents has been done by Helen Fisher; see her book *Anatomy of Love: A Natural History of Mating, Marriage, and Why We Stray.* Another look into the varieties of love, the chemistries they produce, as well as the best guide for making love last, can be found in Pat Love's (her real name!) *Hot Monogamy.*

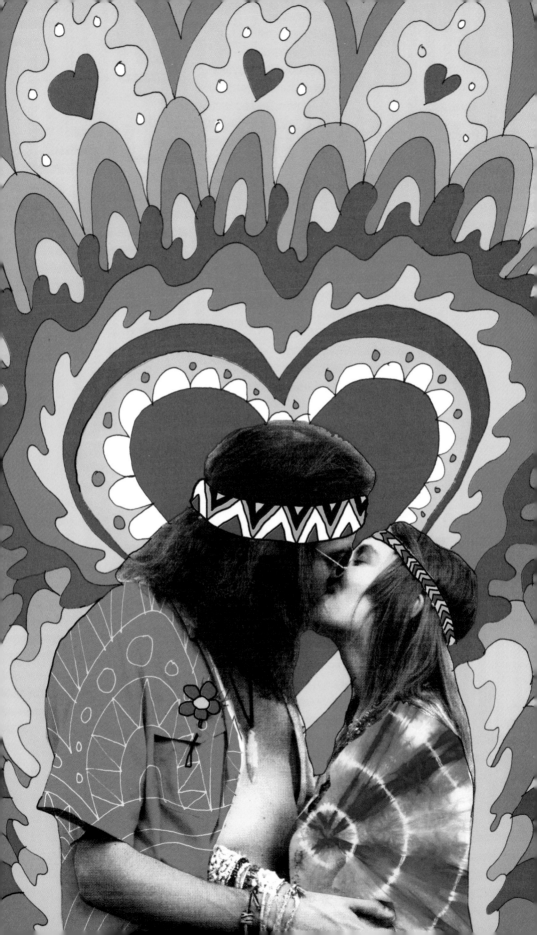

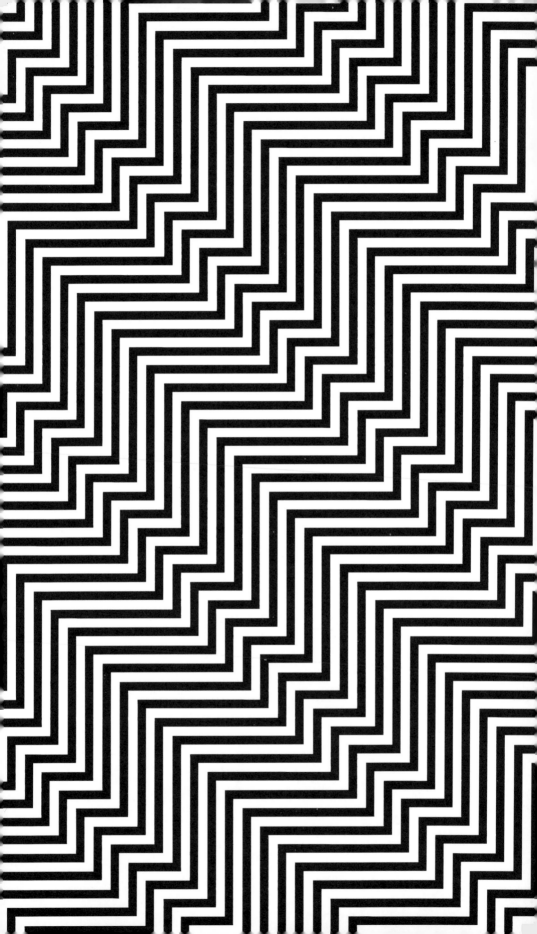

CHAPTER 3

NEGATIVE TECHNIQUES

Many of the following states are painful, emotionally or physically (or both). It is not recommended that one seek out such states, but they are nevertheless a part of the human experience and create unique modes of consciousness. Some of these are states we all experience (paranoia, suffering, pain), while others are experienced by only a select few (psychosis, demonic possession). If you do find yourself slipping too far into one of these negative states, please consult entries such as Meditation (No. 14) and Alterations of breathing (No. 20) to bring yourself back, or seek professional help.

· ·

40 Suffering

Suffering brings about transformation.

Suffering does as much to change the life of human beings as almost anything else. Most of us do not like to suffer; those who do seek it with a passion and explore its every contingency.

Suffering forces us to reassess our position, goals, ways, value, worth, and direction. Suffering brings about transformation. Suffering forces change.

When we are suffering mentally, we are irritated and incomplete. But this suffering, this incompleteness, can be the impetus to finding a new situation for ourselves. Suffering demands relief, new environments, new supports. Physical suffering is characterized by pain and often demands that "new environment" called death.

· ·

41 Pain

A universal experience that increases and dulls awareness.

P ain is any system's resistance to a stimulus. Everyone has and will continue to experience pain. The intensity of the pain experienced will be modulated by the degree of resistance with which a system encounters the pain-producing stimuli.

This systemic production of pain through resistance is fully revealed during activities like Massage (No. 144) or Rolfing (No. 139). Whenever muscles are being manipulated to the point of pain, that pain is reduced when one can open up the muscle and let the manipulation proceed.

Some people are truly turned on by pain. This is usually connected, in very complicated ways, to philosophies of self-suffering. Many people experience sexual pleasure through pain, even ecstatic pleasure. There are different types of pain: dull, sharp, quick, long-lasting. Each of these types bring different experiences. Quick, sharp pain brings about an increase in adrenaline and causes shallow breathing, whereas long, dull pain usually promotes listlessness and depression.

Initial pain brings awareness of systemic resistance. Continuous pain dulls awareness.

Further Resources

T he works of the Marquis de Sade are essential. Some of his most important observations are contained in *120 Days of Sodom, Justine, Philosophy in the Bedroom,* and *Juliette.*

42 Forbidden activities

You're not supposed to do that! But what if you did?

K ILL! KILL! KILL! is a mantra that has been used in training some of the armed forces of the United States. The effectiveness of this training is achieved in part because of the thrill of fantasizing about participation in a forbidden activity. Killing is one such forbidden activity. Many soldiers go on to actually kill other human beings; many don't. Nonetheless, the training situation encourages the trainees to fantasize the experience of killing.

Earlier in evolutionary development, killing was an essential part of everyday carnivorous existence. As the evolutionary journey has progressed, social organization has segregated most killing to slaughterhouses and other such institutions, thus removing it from everyday life. What remains is killing usually done by high-powered weapons and crimes of emotion (stabbings and beatings). Crimes committed with guns involve a killer who is already once removed from his prey:

The distance at which all shooting weapons take effect screens the killer against the stimulus situation which would otherwise activate his killing inhibitions. The deep, emotional layers of our personality simply do not register the fact that the crooking of the forefinger to release a shot tears the entrails of another man.
—ON AGGRESSION BY KONRAD LORENZ

Further Resources

E d Sanders chronicles the forbidden activities of Charles Manson and his gang in the book *The Family*.

. . . .

43 Rage

Anger can be good.

We are taught to express our anger but not to express it directly. However, rage, total anger, can be good for us. For example, when a man is criticized by his boss, social convention and fear of job loss demand that he not respond with what he is really feeling, anger. The result of such a situation is usually displacement: The man's wife, relative, or friend is the target for retaliation instead of the boss. Suppressing anger can be dangerous and self-destructive. As with pain, there is an anger threshold that can be tolerated without expression before a breakout is precipitated.

Most of us resist the expression of our anger because we fear our own (albeit imaginary) omnipotent destructive power. Our central catastrophic fantasy is that if we ever got really angry we'd do something terrible, something so unforgivable that we would end up in serious trouble.

A safe way to experiment with anger is to arrange to get angry at a time when you can be alone or with people you trust. Then you can try getting really angry with an inanimate object, say, a pillow, something that you won't hurt and that won't hurt you. Make believe the pillow is your boss, enemy, friend, parent, teacher, child, or whoever stirs your wrath, and then let the pillow have the full force of your fury. This can be a means toward both physical release and emotional catharsis. You might find your anger is more manageable than you had allowed yourself to believe.

. . . .

44 Paranoia

They are out to get you!

Are you sure? Can you ever really know? I could have sworn they were talking about *you!* Wasn't that your name just then? . . .

And so it goes; sometimes, it seems, forever. In 1963, Laura Archer Huxley brought out a very fine little book containing some simple but profound recipes for experiencing the fullness of being alive. The only problem was the title: *You Are Not the Target.*

The fact is that you *are* the target! The entire universe is a plot that is keeping you alive. Keep in mind that for every intricate scheme that you know about, someone, somewhere, is plotting something even more heinous; and the focus of the plot is you.

What was that noise? Are they whispering? Who's there?

Positive paranoia

Most paranoia concerns delusions of persecution, but positive paranoia exhibits delusions of grandeur. This kind of paranoia is often confused with telepathy and mind reading. You're driving down the highway on February 2, 2022, at 2:02 in the afternoon and you know that the car in front of you will have a license plate with seven twos in it and will be carrying two passengers. And because two is your lucky number, you know that today is the day for you to realize all of your dreams. Everything that happens to you is part of a benefic plot, a grand scheme so marvelous that it's hard for you to believe it's happening to you.

. . . .

45 Panic

Let it all go. Flip out.

All of your catastrophic expectations just came true. There is nothing you can do about it. How can you keep calm at a moment like this? The only thing left to do is to panic: utterly and completely.

It's often the perfect way to handle a situation. If someone else is around, then they become the helper who takes care of you. If there's cause for true panic on your part, they'll enjoy taking care of you. It will keep them from panicking.

Don't indulge yourself in panic when you're alone.

. . . .

46 Psychosis

An intolerable reality.

Psychosis includes hallucinations, delusions, severely disorganized thoughts and behaviors, and other conditions often referred to as madness. Society thinks of psychosis in an extremely negative way. This view protects society from the potential harm of psychotics, such as those with schizophrenia, but does little to aid the psychotic. Often the institutionalization of a psychotic fixes only the patient's psychotic behavior. The theories of R. D. Laing, David Cooper, Aaron Esterson, and others have suggested that madness may be the only possible adaptive response to what the psychotic believes to be an intolerable or unmanageable situation. Laing set up an institution that he called a "blow-out center," where people could receive alternative treatment for psychotic experiences.

The usual treatment for psychosis is hospitalization and medication. The increasing reliance on pharmacological mood manipulation often fails to get to the root of the emotional component of psychosis. At Laing's center an individual was encouraged to work through feelings of madness without being drugged. Often such behavior as shouting and infantile regression was nurtured so as to allow the patient to be able to have some experience of their own sickness. By using this approach, Laing believed that a psychotic might then be able to see the situation with greater clarity and change their response from psychosis to other, alternative forms of behavior.

Each a fuse to set you off . . . If I could turn you on, if I could drive you out of your wretched mind, if I could tell you I would let you know.
—THE POLITICS OF EXPERIENCE BY R. D. LAING

Further Resources

The works of R. D. Laing, especially *The Divided Self, The Politics of Experience, Self and Others,* and *Knots* are most enlightening reads. All of the books comment on, discuss, and make suggestions about the psychotic experience. For a contemporary look at the work of Laing, see Michael Guy Thompson's *The Legacy of R. D. Laing.* Thompson also runs a Facebook group, "R. D. Laing Symposium in the Twenty-First Century," which features events and updates on his work.

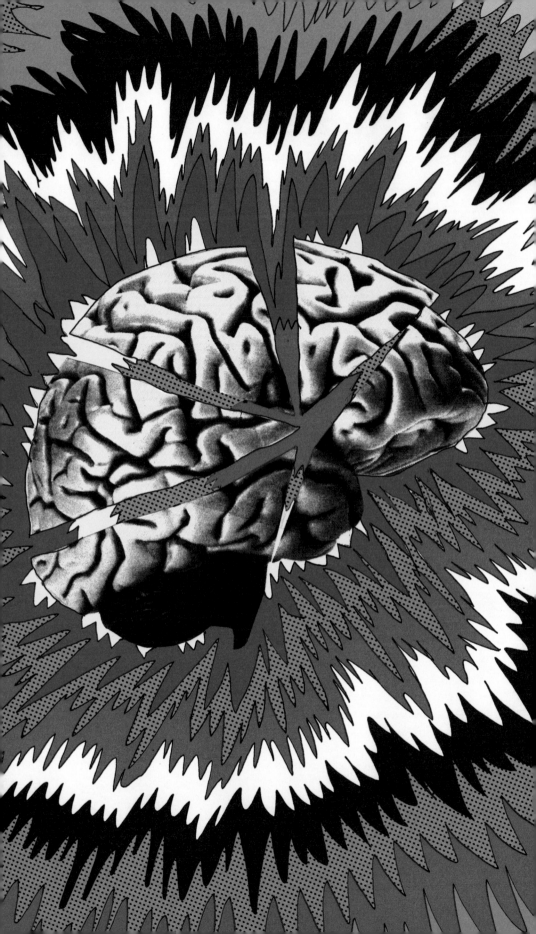

• •

47 Amnesia

Forgetting through trauma or trance.

Amnesia is the experience of losing a portion or the whole of one's memory. It is usually connected with a fight-or-flight process. That is, one experiences trauma, and in an attempt to block its damaging effects, the memory of the event and possibly the events leading up to and following it are totally lost to recall. This often results in lapses of identity.

While most cases of amnesia are brought about by brain injury, you can try to achieve this state via a safer route: Hypnosis (No. 143). Aldous Huxley was able to produce amnesia experiences at will by inducing a light trance. This led to his experiencing selective rather than total amnesia. One example was when he induced a light trance and sat in his armchair. The mailman came, rang Huxley's doorbell, and delivered a special delivery letter. When Huxley's wife returned later, found the letter, and questioned him concerning its arrival, Huxley had no memory of what had transpired. He was able to do this in a variety of different situations. He found that when he attempted to evoke total amnesia he found himself in a deep trance and thereby curtailed in physical activities.

Further Resources

Huxley describes his experiences in Charles Tart's book *Altered States of Consciousness.*

• •

48 Exhaustion

The state of a body and mind depleted.

Exhausting and depleting one's resources brings about altered states of consciousness. True exhaustion often causes physical collapse, hallucinations, apparitions, etc. Often present are feelings of disorientation and tension. Most people experience exhaustion because of overwork. Other ways to bring on an exhausted state are Fasting (No. 57) and Sleep deprivation (No. 58).

• •

49 Delirium of high fevers

A naturally occurring altered state.

Although many people run very high fevers during illnesses and still do not experience delirium, others do so at temperatures as low as 102°F.

One young boy who became delirious with scarlet fever ran a temperature in excess of 104°F for almost two weeks. He began to speak to his parents as though he were wandering through a dream. He did not recognize them, and he seemed to be talking about a peculiarly personal world of his own. He complained that the objects he touched, the sheets and tissues, the thermometer, hurt him and felt like pins and needles.

His sense of size was distorted. Things that he thought were small, like his toys, seemed as big as the whole room, while things that he thought of as large, like his father, seemed to him very tiny. He often responded to voices that only he could hear. Another perceptual distortion was in his experience of time. His mother would leave him alone for five minutes and he would think that she had been gone hours, while at other times, hours were kaleidoscoped into mere seconds.

Though not everyone who experiences delirium goes through visual, auditory, tactile, and time-flow hallucinations, these perceptual alterations are part of many deliriums.

Further Resources

Hudson Hoagland describes his wife's delirious fever experiences in *The Voices of Time* (edited by J. T. Fraser).

· ·

50 Epileptic seizures

The ecstasy and agony of possession.

The convulsive brain-initiated seizures of epilepsy are one of the purest forms of possession. Sometimes the victim of the seizure is not conscious or aware in any way of what is happening to them. Other times, it is an ecstatic, mind-altering, and memorable state.

There are several kinds of epileptic seizures that involve altered states. For example, absence, or "petit mal," seizures, result in a loss of consciousness for only several moments, often not noticed by those witnessing the person experiencing the seizure. The most common type of seizure, a partial or "focal onset aware" seizure, is often accompanied by twitching, nausea, sensory hallucinations, and strange feelings like sudden joy or fear or even déjà vu.

Oliver Sacks, in his book *Hallucinations*, devotes a chapter ("The Sacred Disease") to the various states of consciousness experienced by those who undergo epileptic seizures. He describes the seizure experiences of several patients with epilepsy, including one woman who does not want her seizures to continue but who, nonetheless, describes them as a portal to other forms of consciousness.

Sacks refers to French neurologist Theophile Alajouanine, who observed that the novels and writings of Fyodor Dostoyevsky were influenced by his epileptic seizures, changing from the earlier realistic novels to the later more mystical novels. Dostoyevsky himself greatly valued his seizures. From his personal recollection of one such experience:

> The air was filled with a big noise and I tried to move. I felt the heaven was going down upon the earth and that it had engulfed me. I have really touched God. He came into me myself, yes God exists, I cried, and I don't remember anything else. You all, healthy people . . . can't imagine the happiness which we epileptics feel during the second or so before our fit. . . . I don't know if this felicity lasts for seconds, hours or months, but believe me, for all the joys that life may bring, I would not exchange this one.

Further Resources

See Oliver Sacks, *Hallucinations,* and T. Alajouanine, "Dostoiewski's epilepsy."

• •

51 Migraines

Hallucinations for the price of pain.

M igraines are recurring, severely painful headaches that are usually preceded by visions of patterns or other kinds of hallucinations, e.g., smells, distortions of body shape, etc. Usually migraines are experienced in a localized area of the head. This localization takes place because migraines mostly occur only in either the left *or* the right cerebral hemisphere, though there have been people who experience migraine headaches in both hemispheres of the brain.

Just prior to the onset of a migraine, a specific visual pattern appears. It is often in the form of a sweeping arc or of a honeycomb design; most of the patterns formed are hexagonal, though some are formed by zigzag lines. Geometric patterns are also common.

Oliver Sacks, who himself suffered from migraines from the age of three or four on, sees the patterns in migraine visions as possibly representing the electrical activity of collections of nerve cells, a visual manifestation of the inner workings of our consciousness. "The hallucinatory forms are, in this way, physiological universals of human experience. . . . The geometrical hallucinations of migraine allow us to experience in ourselves not only a universal of neural functioning but a universal of nature itself."

Further Resources

S ee Whitman Richards's "The Fortification Illusions of Migraines" in *Scientific American,* May 1971, and *Hallucinations* by Oliver Sacks. For those who have never suffered from a migraine, the pain-reliever company Excedrin produced a virtual-reality "migraine simulator" that includes reproductions of typical visual hallucinations. You can download it on their website (excedrin.com) or as an app.

· ·

52 Narcotic withdrawal

The pain and delirium of kicking a habit.

Kicking junk (withdrawing from addiction to heroin or other narcotics) is a special kind of hell. It lasts for seventy-two consecutive hours. Although drugs are required to bring about addiction, it is the very absence of drugs that brings on the state of withdrawal. Withdrawal itself is made more severe when no sedatives or pain killers are available to ease the body pains, sweating, nausea, convulsions, and chills.

Barbiturate addiction is much more severe than heroin addiction, as is its withdrawal. Both the addiction and withdrawal are characterized by hallucinations, delirium, disorganization, and motor dysfunction.

· ·

53 Demonic possession

A curse or a privilege?

To be possessed by the devil: to fly through the nighttime sky, to feel another move your limbs, to feel the other in your mind. To know the other. Not all bad. Not all good. Demons may take you to death or to renewed life.

Many cultures have some possession-like contact with demonic spirits. The actual possession by these spirits comes about through a form of ritualistic cultural hypnosis. Often, the demonic spirits are ancestors or animal spirits. The village elders often speak of these spirits, and demonic possession can be considered a privileged state.

Further Resources

Aldous Huxley's *The Devils of Loudun* treats the subject well. It was also made into a movie. A. H. Neal's *Jungle Magic* and Milo Rigaud's *Secrets of Voodoo* treat other aspects of possession.

54 Brainwashing
Inducing a trance through disorientation.

Contrary to popular opinion, the indoctrination technique called brain-washing, or thought control, does not work very well. It is occasionally effective in short-term situations, but temporary results typically fade away.

The temporary results are attained through the removal of familiar social and behavioral signals and through assaults on one's reality-orienting systems. The methods used include repetition, contradiction, sleep depriva-tion, water deprivation, and control of light and temperature.

When brainwashing is carried out over a long period of time, the inten-sity of the results obtained tends to lessen. But if exposure is for a week or so, it can result in extreme psychotic reactions, total disorientation, and in some cases, the onset of physical illness.

Technically, brainwashing can be called a form of intense hypnosis. The results usually produce a subject who is in a kind of trance. They seem con-fused, and bewilderment colors all of their actions. Their behavior is slug-gish, they speak only when spoken to, and their sentences are incomplete. All of this behavior is the result of the destruction of normal patterns of experience.

Further Resources

William Sargant's *Battle for the Mind* has most of the details and pres-ents them accurately and correctly. John Frankenheimer's highly entertaining film *The Manchurian Candidate* gives an exciting but some-what exaggerated view of the results of brainwashing. See also the works of Robert Jay Lifton and Dr. Robert Duncan in *Project: Soul Catcher*, Volume Two.

55 Self-flagellation
You are the inflictor and the recipient.

Self-flagellation means doing yourself in, beating yourself, trying to cause yourself pain, mutilating your body. One must divide oneself to become the inflictor and the victim; the sadist and the masochist within the same person.

There are many ways to accomplish the deed: hitting, beating, whipping, biting, burning, cutting, ripping, shredding, piercing, sewing, binding, scratching, stretching, tearing, etc.

There are some positive uses of self-flagellation, such as the beating of the body in hot baths in order to stimulate blood circulation.

The Penitente group, near Santa Fe, New Mexico, incorporates self-flagellation into their religious rituals and practices. Members of the group flagellate themselves with tree branches in order to experience religious feelings that will help to cleanse and make them acceptable to God.

Further Resources

Self-flagellation is often thought to be an indication of the close relationship between sadism and masochism. The Marquis de Sade may have been the most famous example of this. Jean Paulhan, in his introduction to de Sade's *Justine,* argues the point that De Sade was projecting himself into his masochistic heroine.

· ·

56 Fire walking

A Greek rite and an altered state.

Fire walking and related acts such as sitting on beds of nails, walking across glass, and so forth are usually performed in a trance.

A good example is the rite of the Anastenaria, held each May in Northern Greece. In this rite, ecstatic fire walkers step out onto red-hot coals. Examination of the soles of their feet shows no burns or other markings one would expect to find on flesh that has just touched fire.

These feats of physiological self-regulation are characteristic of the ecstatic states wherein other internal and external functions are controlled. Often, observers of these phenomena are moved to participate. The results run about half and half. Half participate with no ill aftereffects; half are severely burned, cut, or otherwise injured.

Further Resources

See Loring M. Danforth's *Firewalking and Religious Healing: The Anastenaria of Greece and the American Firewalking Movement* and Dimitris Xygalatas's *The Burning Saints: Cognition and Culture in the Fire-walking Rituals of the Anastenaria.* In Greece, the May festival of Anastenaria features public performances of fire walking. Consult the Greek National Tourist Office for specific details. Also see *Trances* by Wavell, Butt, and Epton.

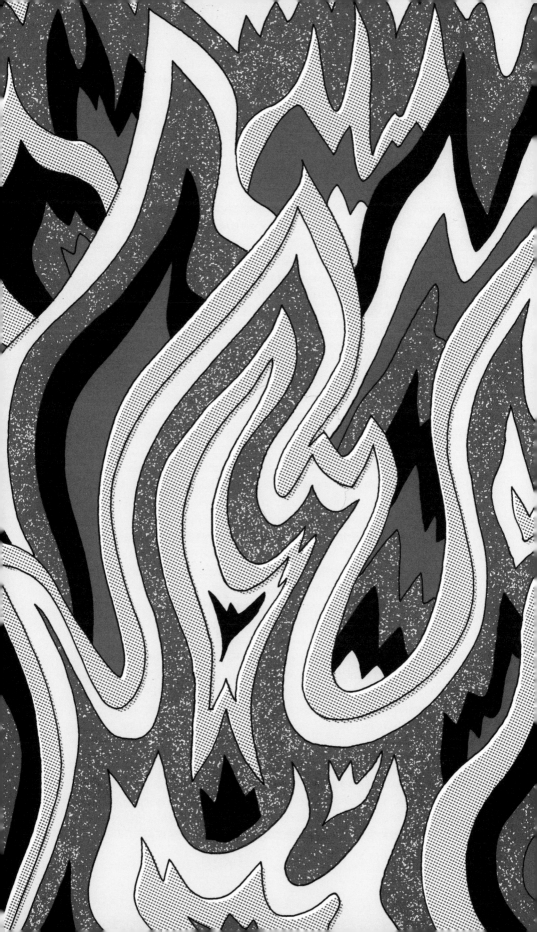

· ·

57 Fasting

Deprivation in one form leads to extraordinary sensations in others.

Fasting can be used in both positive and negative ways. Going without eating can definitely serve the faster by purging and cleansing the body of accumulated poisons and fatty deposits. Most humans carry a good deal of usable energy around with them, energy never used until smaller food intake forces the breakdown of those deposits.

The normal period for cleansing the body is about thirty days. However, this time period varies from person to person, depending on general state of health, body type, and other factors. A cleansing fast is one during which the faster drinks some kind of nutritious liquid (i.e., fruit juice or bouillon) each day. However, infections present in the body will grow during a fast and could become dangerous. There are other potential risks as well. Always consult a doctor and have a complete physical examination before starting a fast.

The negative aspects of fasting are starvation and levels of malnutrition leading to that state. Just how long one has to fast to die depends on the individual and their state of health. Contrary to popular belief, a good fast can go on for many days if the faster is in comfortable, supportive surroundings and has access to medical attention should they need it. The sensation of hunger usually departs after the first three days. It is then that a film forms over the tongue and parts of the inside of the mouth.

While fasting, alterations of a variety of sensory functions occur. Vision can be slightly impaired by susceptibility to illusions and hallucinations. A feeling of seeing things with extraordinarily enhanced color and depth may also spontaneously occur after four days.

The sense of smell, so powerful in animals, is often regained at heightened power in the fasting human being. Odors, usually relegated to background sensory experience, become paramount.

Another phenomenon experienced during long fasts is the "taste hallucination." Here the faster will vividly perceive the tastes of certain foods or spices that he has no real contact with. Many people fast with regularity and find its cleansing characteristics quite beneficial. Some, of course, fast because they have no choice.

Further Resources

Many societies incorporate fasting into seasonal life. A good example is the Hunza group near Pakistan. Renee Taylor discusses their techniques in her book *Hunza Health Secrets*. A good book on the general aspects of the fast is Arnold Ehret's *Guide to Rational Fasting*.

. . . .

58 Sleep deprivation

The delirium of a sleep-starved brain.

Most of us remember some radio DJ who went for several days without sleep as a publicity stunt, or a comedian running the charity telethon for days on end without a nap.

One DJ went without sleep for 230 hours. In 1964, a California high-school student stayed awake for 264.4 hours (11 days and nights) in a controlled experiment. The official record for wakefulness is 449 hours (nearly 19 days), set by a British woman during a rocking-chair competition in 1978. Some have claimed to break this record, but these reports remain unverified, as the *Guinness Book of World Records* no longer officially tracks this category because of the risks involved. Several people have died from lack of sleep. Should you decide to experiment with sleep deprivation, proceed with caution!

After somewhere between 30 and 60 hours, depth perception becomes disturbed; after about 70 hours it becomes difficult to do any normal, easy tasks without errors; after some 90 hours, hallucinations usually set in. After more than 100 hours, the alphabet and other things we "know by heart" become extremely difficult to remember clearly; after 120 hours, delirium; and 150 hours brings about the onset of total disorientation. It is in the later hours that brain waves resemble those of deep-sleep brain waves, even though the nonsleeper might still seem to be awake. Somewhere between the second and fourth day the body begins producing psychochemicals that bear structural resemblance to LSD.

Age most affects the ability to go without sleep. It does not affect the period of sleeplessness; after four days, sleeplessness is hell for anyone. But young people respond better, after completing the sleepless period, than do their elders. The boy who set the 264.4-hour record was only seventeen years old at the time. He needed just 14 hours of sleep after his ordeal, although scientists could still detect aftereffects for ten days after the completion of the project.

Further Resources

Sleep and *Insomnia,* both by Gay Gaer Luce, detail sleep deprivation and provide further references.

· ·

59 Involuntary isolation

The prisoner's cinema.

This usually happens when nature (storms, etc.) or man-made errors (blackouts, elevator failures, etc.) conspire to trap an individual in a place he'd rather not be.

In an elevator, the walls close in after a few hours as the feelings of claustrophobia increase. Situations like this often engender paranoid fantasies, and sometimes psychotic breakdowns.

Blinding snowstorms are often responsible for the hallucinations of trapped drivers or walkers. Men trapped in mines or prisoners in solitary confinement are also known to have experienced altered vision.

· ·

60 Near-death and out-of-body experiences

When the perilous evokes the extraordinary.

Many people who have come close to death, through illness, accident, or other untoward circumstances, report extraordinary experiences, some spiritual in nature, and others in which they seemingly travel outside their bodies.

My first near-death experience (NDE) is illustrative. In the early 1960s, I was riding in a car, driven by my friend. We were on our way to California, coming out of Albuquerque, New Mexico, on the old Route 66. He was speeding, approaching 100 miles per hour, when one of the rear tires blew out. The car wobbled and twisted and turned. As we hit the center divider and crossed into oncoming traffic heading east, I could see everything quite clearly, seemingly in slow motion. The next thing I knew I could feel the shards of glass from what seemed to be the breaking windshield of the car gently caressing my face. It was only when we came to a miraculous safe stop that I realized the glass had not broken and what I had felt were the cigarette ashes spewing out of the ashtray. It was that experience that taught me that the human body can slow down the perception of time, providing a truly altered state of consciousness and time experience.

Often, NDEs involve out-of-body experiences (OBEs). In re-creating OBEs with technology (see No. 250, Simulated body illusions), researchers have discovered that two areas of the brain are disrupted: the hippocampus, which affects our sense of navigation, and the posterior cingulate cortex, which typically creates the sensation of "owning a body."

Oliver Sacks noted: "Neurologically, OBEs are a form of bodily illusion arising from a temporary dissociation of visual and proprioceptive [how we perceive our movement and position] representations—normally these are coordinated, so that one views the world, including one's body, from the perspective of one's own eyes, one's head."

Further Resources

The Near Death Experience Research Foundation (nderf.org) has collected on its website more than four thousand NDEs and other data and resources. *The Handbook of Near Death Experiences* (2009) provides a comprehensive overview of thirty years of research on the subject. For a doctor's investigation of the science of NDEs, see Sam Parnia's *Erasing Death* and *What Happens When We Die?* and Pim van Lommel's *Consciousness Beyond Life: The Science of the Near-Death Experience.* *The Atlantic* published an article covering recent research, "The Science of Near Death Experiences—Empirically Investigating Brushes with the Afterlife," in their April 2015 issue. The Out-of-Body Experience Research Foundation (oberf.org) also includes information and data about OBEs, spontaneous OBEs, NDEs, and deathbed visions.

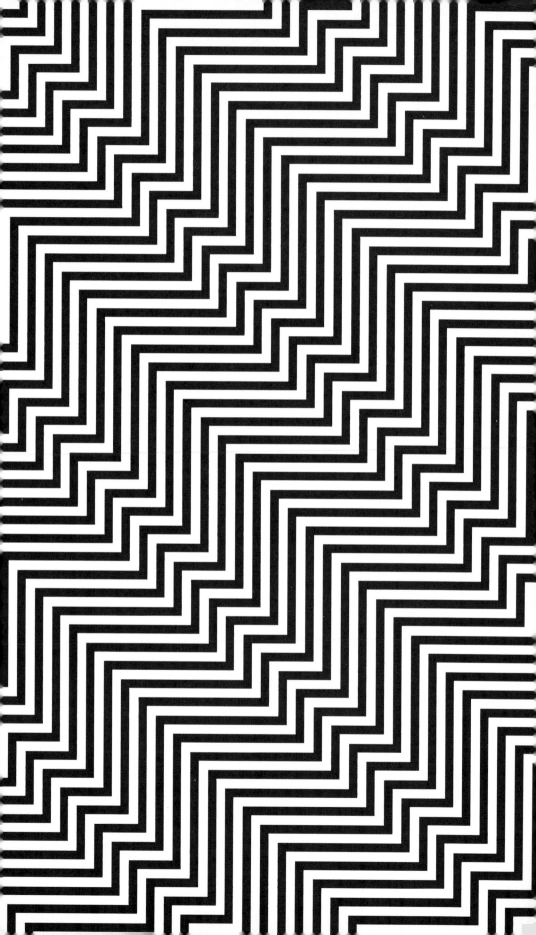

CHAPTER 4

FANTASY, SLEEP, DREAMING, AND SEX

• •

61 Fantasy and daydreaming

Daily escapes into your subconscious.

We all have fantasies and we all daydream. Our society does not sufficiently encourage constructive daydreaming or creative uses of fantasy and the material that fantasy produces.

An important part of the daydreaming process is the ability to let go, to follow the currents of the imagination and allow to emerge whatever will emerge. When we were caught daydreaming at school we were always criticized for not paying attention. Teachers didn't inquire into the content of daydreams. Yet the dreams we dreamt were often quite relevant to the lesson for the day.

Our daydreams and our fantasies contain many keys to our future life. On the creative side, spontaneous material that is germane to our current relationships and projects often becomes available to us in an "idle" daydream. By consciously indulging in fantasy, we can tap hidden resources and release material that might not be available to us in most social situations.

Daydreaming and fantasy have a great advantage in that they are always private activities. There is no way that this privacy can be invaded, short of mindreading.

But daydreaming and fantasy aren't always an entertaining escape. Fritz Perls, the formulator of Gestalt therapy, discussed the use of fantasy as the main way to rehearse for our roles in future activities. This rehearsal can be used to avoid real action and may produce catastrophic expectations which can freeze our ability to truly *be*.

The systematic use of fantasy in psychotherapy has been shown in the work of psychologist R. Desoille. Desoille used a series of daydreams that he felt helped to link the fantasy-creator to their creative collective unconscious. (The collective unconscious was postulated by C. G. Jung in his development of analytical psychology as a repository for universal symbols, or archetypes, that all human beings may draw upon. See Analytical psychology, No. 108.)

Desoille gave his patients six different situations and asked them to act out these situations internally, through their own fantasies. The series of daydreams included:

1 The identification with the sexual symbol: the sword for the male and the ball for the female.

2 A journey to the bottom of the ocean.

3 A journey to the cave of the witch.

4 A journey to the cave of the wizard.

5 A journey to the cave of the mythical beast.

6 The imagining of the patient's own version of the sleeping beauty legend.

Fantasies and daydreams have long been rich source material for stories and tales. Writers often depend on their ability to fantasize within a given, highly structured situation. In this way a plot can be carried through an entire work of fiction.

If you have children and you read them stories, try making up one yourself. Also, ask your children (or nieces, nephews, or friend's children) to tell *you* a story. That way you will be able to see how in touch children are with their daydreams and fantasies.

Further Resources

Psychosynthesis by Roberto Assagioli outlines and details many specific techniques for fantasy development and discusses some of the formulations of Desoille. Yale researcher Jerome Singer has written many articles and books on the subject, including "Ode to Positive-Constructive Daydreaming" in *Scientific American* and the books *Daydreaming* and *Daydreaming and Fantasy.* Psychologist Stanley Kaufman and Carolyn Gregoire's 2015 book *Wired to Create* features an entire chapter on the creative value of daydreaming.

62 Remembering and reverie

Those who do not remember the past are condemned to repeat it.

—GEORGE SANTAYANA

The only place we ever live, in time, is the present. Though the importance of living in the here and now has recently gained more acceptance, many often lose sight of what the here and now is made of: the fabric of our ongoing experience.

Living in the present means not just paying attention to what goes on around us, but realizing that present awareness includes memories of the past and anticipation of the future. Those who fail to live in the present (figuratively, that is; it is impossible to live elsewhere) and attempt to live in the past cannot distinguish between memory as part of present experience and memory as a retreat to a past more real than the present.

Remembering is the essence of knowing. We remember everything, but we are in touch only with selective memories. The reason we do not tap into our full memory-resources is mainly due to selective protective processes in our psychological makeup. It is similar to not actively experiencing all of the data our senses are receiving all of the time. This kind of overloading, like memory overloading, usually proves to be too much to handle. Certain psychedelic drugs as well as some techniques for altering consciousness without drugs stimulate greater contact with both sensory input and memory storage.

Memory is usually activated analogously. That is, when we see something, it reminds us of something else which then activates a memory. This leads to the selective application of memory data to present situations. However, this type of memory use very rarely brings about changed consciousness, except for extraordinarily strong analogous responses, such as the déjà vu sensation. (See Déjà vu, No. 82.)

What will help to alter consciousness is the select and complete use of all memory cues for a given situation. We very rarely take the time out to try to use our memory to completely re-create a special incident or event in our lives. Even when we do, we often neglect very important information regarding the sensory environment at the time of the event, though occasionally this material presents itself spontaneously.

Pick an event about which you have strong feelings and memories. Recreate it with your memory and through the use of controlled reverie, remembering very explicit details that relate to the selected event. This means remembering all of your sensory sensations: what you saw, tasted, heard, smelled, and touched at that time. Be as thorough as possible. When you picture the situation, visualize the furniture or the terrain and recapture the feelings it brought out.

Emotional response is also a tremendous key to memories. If you can recapture the feelings you had in those moments, the experience will be much more realistic.

This technique can be applied to all types of experiences: good, bad, exciting, dull, tense, and excruciating.

Reverie is usually an attempt to recapture the pleasures of the past.

Further Resources

Exercise 5 in *Gestalt Therapy* by Perls, Hefferline, and Goodman deals with ways to get in touch with the forces of remembering. Charles Tart's book *Altered States of Consciousness* includes a number of discussions of remembering during altered states of consciousness. Harmon Bro's *High Play* contain specific instructions for exercises that use reverie to produce altered states of awareness.

. . . .

63 Lullabies

The power of soothing song.

For most of us, lullabies are our first exposure to hypnotic techniques of altering consciousness. The use of repetition (much like mantras) and soothing tones combine to bring about a trance state: sleep.

If a lullaby was used to lull you off to sleep in your childhood, see if it still has any of its magic power left.

Further Resources

In 2013, the journal *The Psychology of Music* published a study on the effects of lullabies on hospitalized children under three years old ("Wellbeing and Hospitalized Children: Can Music Help?"). The *New York Times Magazine* ran a feature, "The Melancholy Mystery of Lullabies," on October 4, 2015. The article discusses Carnegie Hall's long-running Lullaby Project (carnegiehall.org/Lullaby), which also posts its lullabies to SoundCloud (soundcloud.com/carnegiehalllullaby).

64 Sleep

When life becomes unendurable sleep is the escape possible for all men.
—GAY GAER LUCE

We all spend one-quarter to one-third of our entire lives in sleep. Sleep eventually dominates any kind of experience. There is no way to escape it. There is no way to live without it for more than a week or so. (See Sleep deprivation, No. 58.)

Most of us know nothing of who we are and what we do when we are asleep. Considering how much attention we give to various aspects of our waking life, it is astounding how we ignore the life of sleep.

What happens when we go to sleep?

Further Resources

The entire subject of sleep is covered thoroughly and readably by Gay Gaer Luce's two books *Sleep* and *Insomnia*. Both books include copious references and complete bibliographies to aid further work in this area.

65 Dreaming

The mind's playground.

When you go to sleep, you dream. These dream periods are almost always characterized by rapid eye movements (REM) even though the lids remain closed.

More vivid than the finest movies, dreams are great enigmas. All of us dream, even if we don't remember having dreamt. When we don't remember dreaming, it usually means that we awoke from a state of nonrapid eye movement sleep. If we awaken from REM sleep, we should have some memory of the act of dreaming if not of the dream itself.

Dreams can be so vivid that the valves of memory seem to have opened the entire life history of a person, down to the smallest details of smell and touch.
—GAY GAER LUCE

Dreaming is a universally known altered state of consciousness, for we all do many things in our dreams that we might never even "dream" of attempting while awake.

The Dutch physician Frederik van Eeden wrote a study on dreaming that was published in 1913. While there have been many different opinions on how to categorize our dreams that have come since, the impact of van Eeden's work was profound. His paper introduced terms like *lucid dreaming*, which we still use today. Here are Van Eeden's nine experientially distinct types:

1 **THE INITIAL DREAM:** a dream that occurs just after sleep takes over the body, but when the mind is still active.

2 **THE PATHOLOGICAL DREAM:** a dream occurring during high fever or other disturbed states.

3 **THE ORDINARY DREAM.**

4 **THE VIVID DREAM:** a dream that leaves lasting impressions of a vivid nature with the dreamer.

5 **THE SYMBOLIC DREAM OR MOCKING DREAM:** dreams of an occult or "demoniacal" nature.

6 **THE DREAM-SENSATIONS DREAM STATE:** a dream where the normal images and events do not occur, but the dreamer awakens knowing he or she has been occupied with one person, one place, etc.

7 **THE LUCID DREAM:** a dream where the dreamer is aware that he or she is dreaming, though this awareness does not interfere with the dream, but rather augments it.

8 **THE DEMON DREAM:** a dream nightmare where the demon causing or perpetrating the dream action is seen clearly.

9 **THE WRONG WAKING-UP DREAM:** a dream where the dreamer dreams that he or she has awakened, only to discover that the waking up is only part of the dream.

In his summary of van Eeden's work, Charles Tart added another dream: *the high dream.* In the high dream, the dreamer is aware that he is dreaming and is also aware that he is experiencing an altered state of consciousness, much like the kind brought on by taking psychedelics or by using certain techniques described in this book.

The next few entries discuss ways in which one can experience the special states of dreams more fully.

Further Resources

Gay Gaer Luce's book *Body Time* provides detailed data and discussion. Tart's section on dreaming in *Altered States of Consciousness* is one of the best in the book. *The International Journal of Dream Research: Psychological Aspects of Sleep and Dreaming* is a peer-reviewed journal with contemporary research on dreaming. G. William Domhoff, a psychology professor at the University of California, Santa Cruz, and the author of several books on dreaming, runs a website that collects papers on the subject, as well as a Dream Bank cataloging more than twenty thousand dreams (www2.ucsc.edu/dreams).

• •

66 Dream incubation

Writing your own dreams.

There are many factors that influence our dreams. When we sleep during a thunderstorm, we might awaken from a dream in which the last thing experienced was an enormous, ear-filling noise. The first thing to occupy our consciousness upon awakening will be the receding noise from a clap of thunder. What we have done in this case is to incorporate the stimulus into the dreaming experience. That stimulus, to some extent, controlled the dream. A more frequently occurring experience of this type is the incorporation of the sound of an alarm clock.

You do not need to rely on environmental stimuli to influence your dreams. With dream incubation, you can prime yourself to dream of certain themes. A way to control the content of dreaming is to control the stimuli that you are exposed to just before going to sleep. If you carefully examine pictures of galaxies, and think about dreaming about galaxies, chances are that you might have dreams of galaxies and stars. Another way is to induce a self-hypnotic trance and give posthypnotic instructions about dream content while still in the trance.

One interesting area of dream incubation is dream-based problem solving. Many artists and inventors claim to have achieved breakthroughs in their dreams. In one study, researchers primed students to think about a particular homework assignment in their dreams. Half of the students dreamt about the assignment and 70 percent of that group dreamt of a solution to the assignment.

Try an experiment in which you select a problem or scene that you would like to focus on in your dream. Before bed, focus on this problem, set an intention that you will dream about it (say aloud, "I will dream about . . ."). Barrett even recommends placing visual cues on your nightstand.

Further Resources

The study on dreams and problem solving was conducted by Deirdre Barrett, who researches dream incubation at Harvard. See her book *The Committee of Sleep* and visit her website (deirdrebarrett.com).

67 Hypnagogic phenomena

Drowsiness before sleep.

Hypnagogic hallucinations was the term, coined in 1848 by French psychologist Alfred Maury, to describe the visions and activities some people experience in the drowsiness that precedes sleep.

Most people have experienced the hypnagogic state: It is that state of limbo just before you fall asleep where you are neither awake nor asleep. This state is characterized by images, visions, conversations—mentally created events that we do not consciously generate or manipulate. They occur quite spontaneously.

Some people claim that they never experience this phase, while others actively seek it for the free-flowing creative consciousness brought into play during this special drowsiness. Scientists, inventors, artists, and others have reported that they get many of their best ideas during their hypnagogic experiences.

Charles Tart devised a relatively easy way to tap the hypnagogic phenomenon. Lie down on your back and let yourself start to drop off into the hypnagogic state prior to sleep. But keep your arm in the air by bending it at the elbow. This way, when you start to really drop into the state of sleep the muscles of the arm will totally relax, causing the arm to fall. This will wake you up. Then you can start the procedure again, from the beginning. With some practice, you will soon be able to remember what transpires during the hypnagogic state.

Try for yourself. Be aware of what happens to you in the hypnagogic state. It is possible that you might find some interesting images based on your experiences of the day or see your experiences in a new perspective. Or you might suddenly arrive at a solution to a problem that has been disturbing you.

Further Resources

Tart's book *Altered States of Consciousness* includes an entire section devoted to reports on hypnagogic phenomena. In *Hallucinations*, Oliver Sacks includes a chapter, "On the Threshold of Sleep," containing a great deal of material on and insight into hypnagogic and hypnopompic hallucinatory phenomena, as well as quotes from many different people describing their hypnagogic visions and sounds. Sacks notes: "Few phenomena give such a sense of the brain's creativity and computational power as the almost infinitely varied, ever-changing torrent of patterns and forms which may be seen in hypnagogic states."

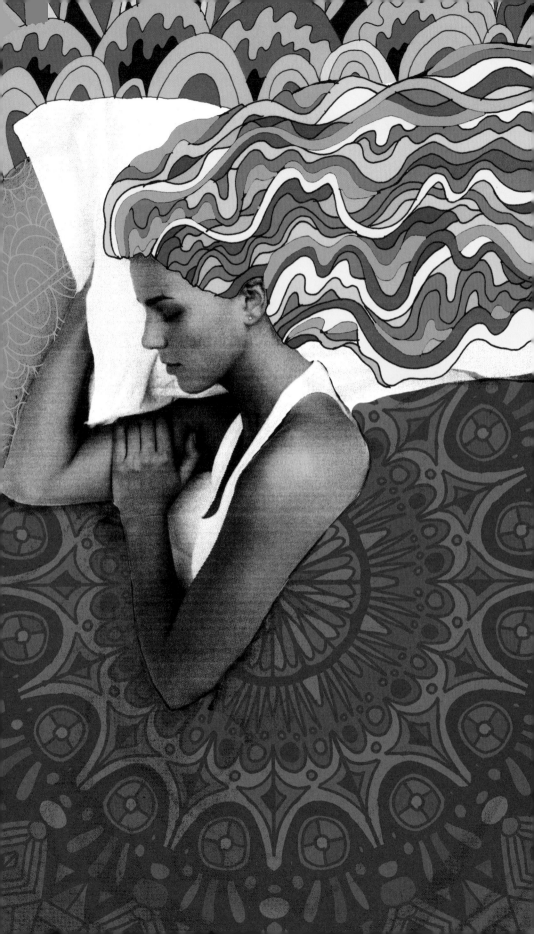

. . . .

68 Lucid dreaming

Being an active participant in your dreams.

An interesting experiment is to attempt to self-program the control of dreams. This would include using not only environmental controls and the programming of presleep stimuli, but would also attempt to raise the level of awareness during the dreaming state. Simple presleep suggestions to the effect that you, as a dreamer, will have lucid dreams, where you are aware that you are dreaming, can be employed.

How else might one reach this state of conscious awareness while dreaming? Here are a few guidelines from *A Field Guide to Lucid Dreaming* by Jared Zeizel, Dylan Tuccillo, and Thomas Peisel:

1   Get accustomed to performing "reality checks." If you find yourself in what seems to be a dream, performing a reality check will be the best way to confirm that you are, in fact, dreaming. Can you poke your finger through the palm of your hand? Do you have your usual number of fingers? When you jump, do you come down? Perform these checks during your waking hours to make them a habit.

2   We experience our most active dreaming in the last two windows of REM sleep in the early morning. You can ensure that you are best primed to actively dream in this state with a strategy that Zeizel et al., refer to as "wake-back-to-bed." Wake up after six hours of sleep, stay awake for twenty minutes, then go back to bed. Doing this wakes up your brain, particularly the left analytical side. Not only are you now primed to enter a peak dream state, but your alert brain will recognize it.

3   If you perform your reality checks and realize you are in fact in a dream, you'll want to prolong your lucidity by moving and interacting with your surroundings. Dream researcher Stephen LaBerge recommends performing a pirouette—by challenging your dream body, you will ground yourself in the dream.

4   Have fun. Once you've stabilized yourself in the dream, it's time to play. Fly. Teleport. Walk through walls. This is a world with no rules. Interact with someone—is it a person with whom you have a conflict during the day? Perhaps you can resolve it in the safe space of the dream.

5   When you do wake up, don't wake up too quickly! Don't open your eyes. Stay focused. Stay still. Try to remember everything that happened in your dream. Then write it down in a dream journal.

By becoming more present in your dreams, you will be more present in your waking life as well.

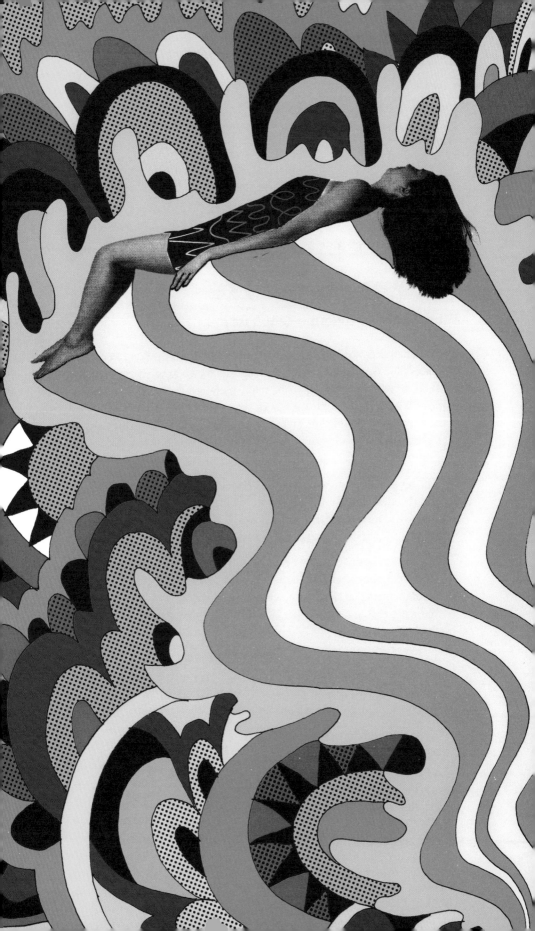

Further Resources

See *A Field Guide to Lucid Dreaming: Mastering the Art of Oneironautics* by Dylan Tuccillo, Jared Zeizel, and Thomas Peisel. Also *Exploring the World of Lucid Dreaming* by Stephen LaBerge and Howard Rheingold.

. . . .

69 Dreams applied to waking life

What can our dreams teach us?

Freud and others believed that dreams were a key to the past. Perls and others held that dreams were an existential message about the present. For more than four thousand years, many men have believed that dreams bear messages about the future. There are various applications of dreams to the activities of waking life. I will briefly discuss two of them. Fritz Perls, in Gestalt psychotherapy, particularly liked to work with patients on their dreams:

> I believe that in a dream, we have a clear existential message of what's missing in our lives, what we avoid doing and living, and we have plenty of material [in the dream] to re-assimilate and re-own the alienated parts of ourselves.

> In Gestalt Therapy we don't interpret dreams. We do something much more interesting with them. Instead of analyzing and further cutting up the dream, we want to bring it back to life. And the way to bring it back to life is to re-live the dream as if it were happening now.

> . . . Write the dream down and make a list of all the details in the dream. Get every person, every thing, every mood, and then work on these to become each one of them. Ham it up, and really transform yourself into each of the different items.

> Next, take each one of these different items, characters, and parts, and let them have encounters between them. Write a script. [Not literally, but figuratively: provide motivation and action.]

Besides using improvised psychodrama techniques à la *Rashomon* (with each character having his own version of the same event), Perls also used a short-cut; this involved finishing what was left unfinished in the action of the dream. An example: if the dream involves a character who is about to start an action, but the dream ends before any action is initiated, Perls would have the dreamer, when working on the dream, complete the action while reliving it in the here and now.

Perls believed that the dream has a direct relevance to the dreamer's present life situation. He felt this was true also of repetitive dreams. Since he used all the elements of a given dream in the analysis of the dream, Perls could work easily with complete dreams, unfinished dreams, and even dream fragments.

Unknown to Perls was the fact that a community has existed for roughly five thousand years that puts many of his theories of dream work to daily, community-wide use. This group is the Achuar tribe of the Ecuadorian Amazon. Also known as the "Dream People of the Amazon," the tribe wakes every day at 4 a.m. for "wayusa" or "dream sharing." Believing that every person's dreams belong to the community, they interpret one another's dreams and are responsible for resolving conflicts in one another's nightmares.

Further Resources

The material from Perls comes from his books *Gestalt Therapy Verbatim* and *In and Out the Garbage Pail*. The practices of the Achuar were explored in an October 2010 *New York Times* feature "Amazon Awakening," as well as the book *A Field Guide to Lucid Dreaming*.

· ·

70 Hypnopompic phenomena
Hallucinations upon waking.

Very little is known about that dawn area of our normal sleeping cycle, the time between sleeping and waking. Oliver Sacks contrasts hypnagogic experiences that occur before going to sleep with hypnopompic experiences that take place after sleep and upon awakening. While hypnagogic hallucinations typically seem more distant—seen through closed eyes, "in their own imaginative space," and without a physical presence—hypnopompic hallucinations "are often seen with open eyes, in bright illumination; they are frequently projected into external space and seem to be solid and real."

A friend has reported that he is able to spend several hours of his sleeping cycle, on some days, actively experimenting with the hypnopompic state. In this experimentation he allows himself to become aware of being awake enough to manipulate his state of consciousness, but not so much as to destroy his ability to resume a state of sleep wherein dreams could develop. In this way he is able to experience very vivid dreams.

His semicontrol of the hypnopompic state allows him to remember many of these vivid dreams. It also enables him, on occasion, to awaken from a dream, hypnopompically perceive that the dream is incomplete or unfinished, return to the sleep state, and reenter the dream. He is not always able to use hypnopompic awareness to control his dreaming, but he reports that the shifting back and forth between dreaming-sleep, hypnopompic awareness, and waking often brings about feelings of having had a very complete night's sleep.

If you want to try this kind of hypnopompic experiment, it will be best to stay still upon awakening, with eyes closed. Let your state of sleep envelop you, even if you briefly awaken. This may not work for all, but trying to master and play with the back and forth of sleep, dreaming, and awakening can yield a delightful state.

Further Resources

Hallucinations by Oliver Sacks, chapter eleven, "On the Threshold of Sleep." Deirdre Barnett's *The Committee of Sleep* discusses how some of the creative epiphanies many attribute to dreams may in fact occur during hypnopompic states.

· ·

71 Sunbathing
Where sleep phenomena meet the kiss of the sun.

Sunbathing offers the unique opportunity to experience and manipulate a variety of states of consciousness while still being a social, even public animal.

Sunbathing allows hypnagogic and hypnopompic phenomena to develop at a variety of different intervals, depending on how much time one spends. The physical changes brought on by exposure to the sun—dehydration, excessive sweating, phosphene stimulation (when the sun is directly in line with the closed eyes), and the fatigue brought on by exposure—make sunbathing potentially a fine time for playing with altered states of consciousness.

After some exposure to the sun, the skin begins to dry out and feels tight and tingling. At the same time certain areas of the body—the armpits, the groin, the face, the scalp—begin to give off perspiration. The free flow of these bodily juices is almost like a consciousness "lubricant" when combined with the feeling of heat on the genitals. Sunbathing is exciting.

72 Floating

The release of weightlessness.

The floating experience is very similar to the sunbathing experience. The extra element is, of course, the water on which you are floating. Such contact with the water can totally alter the tactile, olfactory, and auditory self-perceived environment.

Especially in saltwater, where floating can be done easily and for long periods of time, the sound of the lapping waves, the odor of the salt air, and the all-enveloping feelings of the surrounding water combine to create very special feelings.

Add to these factors the sun, the slipping into and out of various states of sleep, dream, and hypnagogic and hypnopompic awareness, and you have another instance where turning on can be achieved in a very social situation.

The undulating water laps at your body as the tide pulls the sea back and forth, in and out. The sea massages your body with its coolness as the sun warms both the air and your body. Your buoyancy carries you off into a personal, erotic state of consciousness.

Further Resources

See Sensory deprivation (No. 193), which discusses floating in sensory deprivation tanks.

73 Sex

What turns you on?

Sex is the means of altering consciousness that almost everyone has had the pleasure of knowing. Sex can bring about intense states and feelings, including a sense of unity and oneness, a sense of absorption as well as changes in one's perceptions of space, time, and the experience of self. Different people have different sexual pleasures, different tastes, different fantasies that will sexually turn them on. Each of us has the right to enjoy sex.

Sex therapist Tammy Nelson has noted that sexual fantasies are an excellent technique for finding out what turns you on. You can fantasize about anything sexual that makes you feel good, no matter how outrageous that might seem. Indulge your wildest fantasies, and know that just thinking something, no matter how realistic your fantasy might be, cannot hurt you, in and of itself. And a good fantasy has the potential to excite you, to turn you on to new, personal sexual possibilities.

And to fulfill your sexual potential you will have to allow yourself to discover your own sexual depth. Maybe most of the time you are shy, quiet, and passive, but part of you yearns to be more aggressive, stimulating, exuberant, and alive. Perhaps you have never experienced your own sexual gentleness or caring. All of these roles and many more are open and available to you.

We are living in a wonderful era of increased adventurousness and intimacy in expressing our sexuality. One of the biggest changes in contemporary sexuality is the role of women in sex. Women are often now more in charge, driving sexual decisions made in the bedroom and elsewhere. As a result of the increased role of women in sex, orgasm has become more important, for all sexual partners.

What's more, there's now better communication about wants, desires, and needs from partners and participants: a participatory eroticism. Let's talk about sex, baby!

And there is now more freedom in sex, more license to experiment, to innovate, to try new and different things. More people are willing to indulge, to share their fantasies, to act out new and different roles. This can enable you to overcome fears and anxieties and to embrace new possibilities for sexual activity and pleasure.

For some this can mean extremes, like exploration of new roles, even dominance and submission, perhaps even to experiment with pain in the context of sex. For some, to hurt or be hurt can be a source of giving and receiving pleasure.

Experiment with yourself. Try out everything. See how you feel. Be sexy with yourself . . . be sexy with another. Be sexy.

Further Resources

Getting the Love You Want by Tammy Nelson is a thought-provoking guide to sexual possibilities. Guide to Getting It On by Paul Joannides provides a thorough, almost nine-hundred-page guide to everything sexual. Even though their evasively pedantic language makes them difficult to read, both books by William Masters and Virginia Johnson—Human Sexual Response and Human Sexual Inadequacy—are excellent collections of data on sex. W. Reich's The Function of the Orgasm is excellent and is readably expanded upon by Alexander Lowen's Love and Orgasm.

74 Prolonged sexual intercourse

Coalesce to a cosmically deep climax.

The longer the better. After ten or fifteen minutes sexual intercourse becomes more interesting, as your movements become more subtle. After a half hour or so, as with most other repetition-based phenomena, your consciousness will begin to change. Sensations begin to take on new ecstatic aspects as the one-hour mark is approached. Now only the sexual-body energy-environment exists. Now sensations blend and coalesce. Letting go to orgasmic climax is pyrotechnic, possibly divine, cosmically deep.

The man's problem with prolonged sexual intercourse is finding the technique that will help avoid a premature conclusion. Techniques include changing the speed of your movements, stopping movement short of orgasm, talking, changing your breathing, taking a series of shallow breaths, shouting or screaming, opening your eyes, thinking about nonsexual things until the crest of approaching orgasm passes, biting your lip, counting, or holding your breath. The woman may choose to hold off her orgasm or she may go ahead and have any number.

After a certain time, which will vary from couple to couple, a threshold will be reached. At this point orgasm isn't just around the corner, and the lovemaking seems to take over body, mind, and spirit. Then prolonged intercourse may proceed indefinitely.

75 Orgasm

To be purged and completed, spent and fulfilled.

The human sexual orgasm can be the most ecstatic, most exciting experience in life, and certainly is a time-honored way to alter consciousness and leave this world.

Wilhelm Reich was the first to systematically and scientifically examine the human sexual orgasm. His work has recently been carried on by followers Alexander Lowen and Stanley Keleman. Reich felt that: "The severity of any kind of psychic disturbance is in direct relation to the severity of the disturbance of genitality." He postulated that a patient's emotional problems were directly related to their ability to achieve full genital response, or orgasm.

Reich's work also defined two types of orgasm: genital orgasm and full body orgasm. Genital orgasm results from a build-up of energy resulting from the stimulation of the glans penis or the clitoris. When this energy builds up to a certain point, the orgasm occurs.

But there is the possibility of a fuller, more complete, most satisfying orgasmic experience. This is the full body orgasm. Keleman describes this for the male:

> The orgasm can also be triggered from inside, from the pelvic cavity, and if you allow the excitement to run back in the penis . . . and re-excite and flood the whole body, then the whole body is capable of discharging, not just the penis.

In the buildup to full orgasm, sensations of excitement fill your body, you begin to rhythmically move your pelvis, and then you lose control and no longer consciously direct your actions. Your pelvis begins to move forward and back. You can feel the sexual energy flowing freely through your body. You are charging and discharging. You are purged and completed, spent and fulfilled at one and the same time.

What frightens many people about a full body orgasm is the loss of control, the letting go: If they have a full orgasm they will lose control and lose their grip on reality. When control is surrendered, your body takes over, takes charge. It is this experience of letting go and being completed by orgasm that enables us to taste what the ecstatics, mystics, and shamans have been reporting for centuries.

Further Resources

Wilhelm Reich believed that a true sign of a patient's health was the ability to achieve a full body orgasm. His study of the dynamics of orgasm are contained in *The Function of the Orgasm*. Part of the same work is summarized and extracted in *Wilhelm Reich: Selected Writings*. Alexander Lowen writes about orgasm in his *Love and Orgasm* and *Pleasure*. The Stanley Keleman quote comes from his *Sexuality, Self & Survival*. There are several articles detailing the recent rise of Orgasmic Meditation (OM). See the *Atlantic*'s April 2014 article "The Rise of the Pro-Orgasm Movement" or the *New York Times* March 2009 article "The Pleasure Principle."

76 Nudity
Accept your naked body.

W e are born into this world without clothes. Immediately after birth our bodies are clothed, whether environmental conditions demand clothing or not. From then on, our social conditions require that we wear clothing and pay inordinate attention to its style, selection, and maintenance.

After childhood, even the most naive investigation of the unclothed body is frowned upon, and considered to be embarrassing and wrong.

Take time to examine your own body carefully, inside and out. Use mirrors. Look carefully and pay attention to minutiae. Examine your *entire* body, being careful not to overlook anything. Overcome your embarrassment and let your curiosity guide you. Be satisfied.

Walk around your house or apartment nude. Be aware of yourself as a being, without clothes, one who is fully prepared for life. Sense your body and move so that you can feel how your naked body functions free of clothing.

77 Prolonged masturbation
Drive on and find glory.

P rolonged masturbation, or masturbation accompanied by strong emotional content, highly charged fantasies, and the like, can produce altered states of consciousness. The state is very similar to certain trance states, including those induced through hypnosis.

If, after the orgasm (and a small rest), a man continues self-stimulation, he will begin to feel certain changes in his consciousness. Some of these can be due to the fatigue brought on by the exertion of continuing masturbation beyond the energy-releasing orgasm. Others have to do with the inner changes of physio-chemistry brought about by the increase in adrenaline and other hormonal secretions.

In the female, the changes may be more subtle. The fact that no seminal ejaculation occurs means more energy may be available to the female system. Multiple orgasms are possible and delightful.

For either men or women, the altered state of consciousness produced through prolonged masturbation requires a dedication to purpose over and above feelings of exhaustion or the waning erotic interest in the by-now satisfied sexual urge.

Prepare an erotic setting: Turn your phone off, dim the lights, or light a candle. After orgasm, when interest would normally flag, evoke erotic fantasies and images.

For some, fantasies and the promise of an altered state of consciousness will be enough motivation to go on beyond exhaustion and orgasmic satisfaction. Others may use techniques such as pornographic pictures, videos, or literature or perhaps some sexual implement, like a dildo.

The ability to relax, let go, and experience the erotic feelings still present within you, even after a series of orgasms, is difficult but most rewarding. Drive on and find glory.

Further Resources

To my knowledge the only essay that deals with this phenomenon is R.E.L. Masters's "Sexual Self-Stimulation and Altered States of Consciousness," which appears in a volume that Masters edited, entitled *Sexual Self-Stimulation.*

• •

78 Orgiastic or corybantic dancing

Dance to orgasm.

Dance until you drop. Dance as sex, as animal, as energy. Dance until the "you" is lost. Dance and spin and jump and be. Dance to abandon. Dance to orgasm.

Dancing allows you to feel all of the parts of your body as they unite and come together and stretch in all directions. Dancing lets you express inner feelings and feel inner expressions as with no other type of movement.

Dancing by yourself will give you insight into the many ways that you may manifest your being. The only partner that you will have to satisfy will be your own projections, your own feelings. You will be allowed to do things you might never dare reveal to a partner. It will be your dance.

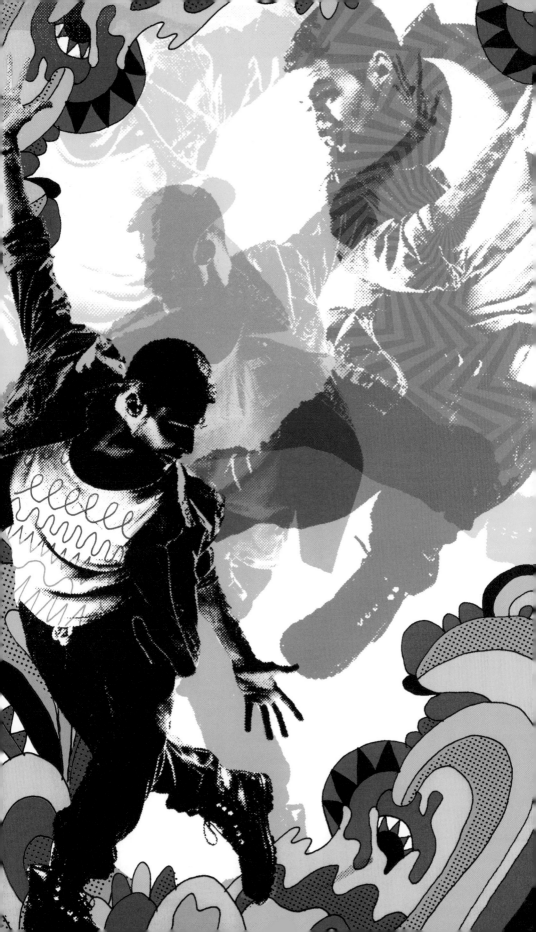

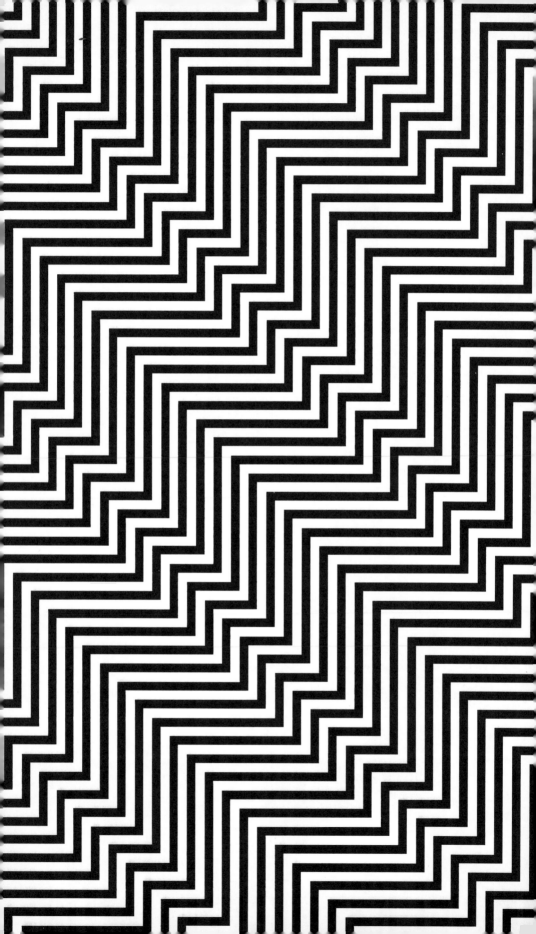

CHAPTER 5

EVERYDAY LIFE

79 Zen morning laugh

Where meditation meets mirth.

This technique was taught to me by the late philosopher Alan Watts, who learned it from a Japanese Zen master in California. The Zen master does this every morning as a form of meditation. He indicates that it accomplishes something similar to rigorous *zazen* without the aching legs that usually attend several hours of sitting.

The gist of the technique is to arise each morning and assume a standing position. Put your hands on the back part of your hips, with your palms faced upward. Now, begin to laugh. Keep laughing. Let your laughter feed off itself and propel itself through your body and out. Laugh fully and completely for a few minutes. When it feels comfortable, stop laughing.

This is a great way to start the day. After a Zen morning laugh, you're ready for anything.

Further Resources

See the *Book of Highs* YouTube playlist for a video of Alan Watts giving a detailed description and demonstration of this technique.

80 Impressions are food

The nourishment of sensation.

When we feel hungry we satisfy this need by seeking nourishment: food. We eat and fulfill the need for several hours.

But edible food is not the only type of nourishment our selves seek. We also seek the nourishment of impressions, stimulation, excitement.

We don't think of the seeking and receiving of impressions as being the same process as that involved in satisfying food hunger. But in many ways the processes are similar.

Experiments with both animals and children have shown that those exposed to more impressions, more stimulation, and more attention are the ones who make a healthy adaptation to the environment and develop their senses. Infants who are deprived of attention, impressions, and stimulation are often deficient in natural growth. Some become impaired in their development.

Boredom is an instructive example; it begins with the manifestation of restlessness. After a while the restlessness might be translated into nervous energy or into idle play (twiddling thumbs, etc.). By the time the experience of ennui has set in, one could be driven to distraction. And that is the point, *to be driven*. And to have that drive results in distraction. By this I mean that impressions and stimulation can then be sought out and replace, or feed, the needs earlier experienced as boredom.

If, when you feel bored, you can stay with the experience without trying to change it; if you can really feel your boredom, you will see what a hungry state it is.

81 Sensory reminiscence

Remembering tastes, smells, sights, sounds, and feelings.

Sensory reminiscence is very close to what I described when I spoke of true remembering (see Remembering and reverie, No. 62). I call attention to it again because we have opportunities to put sensory reminiscence to work every day, with powerful results.

We are constantly referring to our past experiences to help us sort out and make sense of current sensations and events. But we most often stop short of really *experiencing* some of the keen elements of our past experience.

A good place to start is with bacon. Can you remember it right now? Can you see it as it lies in the pan, cold? Can you see it as the heat begins to curl the edges of each strip? Can you smell the heavy odor as the smoke from the bacon rises out of the pan, permeating the kitchen? Perhaps you can think of some other predominant, unmistakable memories. What about being alone in a field? If it was a pretty day there are all sorts of sensory data to go back to, to make into a collage for present appreciation.

These trips into our past experiences can help to make our senses keener and more precise for the present and the future. It is only when we learn to truly put something to use that it will work for us and show us both how to live and how we do live.

82 Déjà vu

Been there. Or have I?

Déjà vu is a French term; the literal translation is "already seen." But it is not quite as simple as having seen something before.

In déjà vu, what is involved is not just a sensory reminiscence but an entire complex of attitude and experience. Déjà vu is being swept up in the feeling that it is the second time around for this particular sequence of life. The feeling is that somewhere, sometime, somehow one has precisely experienced what is happening, and knows what is going to happen next.

What accompanies this feeling is the nagging sensation of not being quite able to tell where, when, or how this past experience was lived. But the feeling of having already lived through it is strong and persistent.

Déjà vu cannot be brought on at will, but it is an experience well worth waiting for.

· ·

83 Synesthesia
Blending of the senses.

S ynesthesia is the mixing of sensory sensations. For example, hearing a sound and, spontaneously, tasting chocolate. Another version of synesthesia can involve perceptual experiences in which seeing a letter or a word evokes the perception of a color. It has been reported that synesthesia is innate: You're born with it. It has also been reported that artists often have experiences of synesthesia, though many others, besides artists, are synesthetes—people who have this mixed perceptual set of experiences.

A 2012 study at the University of Amsterdam attempted to see whether synesthesia can be taught to people who were not born with the ability to cross senses. Though inconclusive, it did offer hope that perhaps future research, or the development of perceptual devices and equipment, might one day enable many more people to experience cross-sensory phenomena.

The mixing of these senses can be expansive, confusing, even both at the same time; a true altered state of awareness.

You can test yourself for synesthesia at synesthete.org. Even if you are not a natural synesthete, there are several ways to try to experience the world from this unique perspective. Israeli artist and jazz musician Michal Levy, who sees colors and shapes as tones and harmonies, created an animated video depicting her synesthetic experience called *Giant Steps* (michalevy.com).

Further Resources

W hether or not you're a synesthete, there are plenty of resources to learn more about the phenomenon. The American Synesthesia Association (synesthesia.info) features research, news, and events. A project studying synesthesia was undertaken at Boston University and a great deal of research and information about synesthesia phenomena can be found on its website (bu.edu/synesthesia/faq/), even though the project has been completed. See also Richard Cytowic's books *The Man Who Tasted Shapes* and *Wednesday Is Indigo Blue: Discovering the Brain of Synesthesia.* For an incredibly detailed dive into synesthesia, consult *The Oxford Handbook of Synesthesia,* edited by Julia Simner and Edward M. Hubbard.

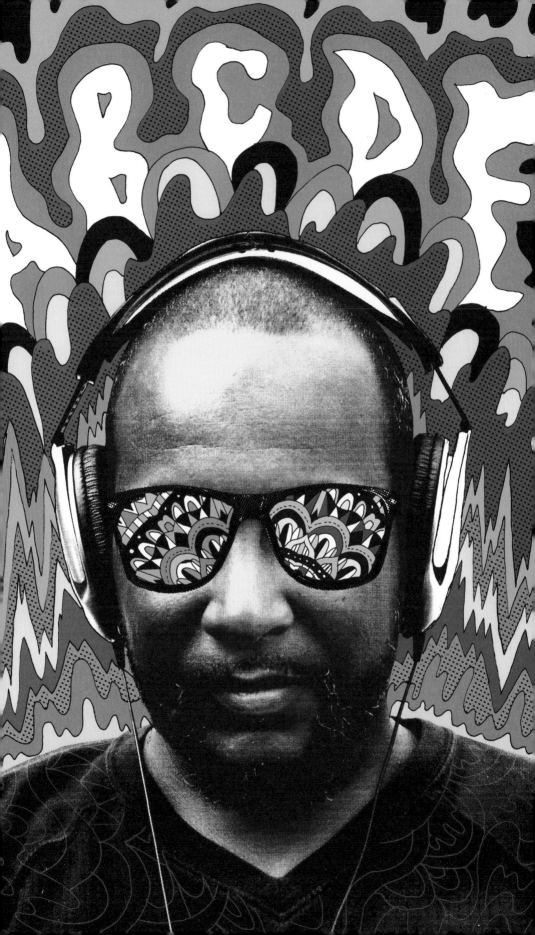

. . . .

84 Seeking
Searching for new ways of being.

Freedom is and must always be at the beginning: it is not an end, a goal to be achieved. One can never be free in the future. Future freedom has no reality, it is only an idea. Reality is what is.
—KRISHNAMURTI, PHILOSOPHER AND SPIRITUAL LEADER

I t is the intangible that we seek most deeply. For many, seeking is all that is worth doing. Seeking becomes an occupation in itself. Sometimes seekers are convinced that seeking is The Way.

In the course of seeking, the seeker may happen upon someone who claims to have found. The seeker may be temporarily impressed, but soon he will resume his search, his life of The Way. The one who has spoken of finding speaks from ignorance, so the true seeker thinks. And his search goes on.

But seeking in itself can also be a revelatory experience. It can be a search for understanding, for values, teachers, helpers, new ways to *be*.

What is sought after in all cases is the self. The end of the search comes when the parts of the self not known to the self are revealed.

. . . .

85 Forgetting
Let it go.

I f we agree that the only constant of life is change, we must loosen our hold on all that is precious to us. If we are to bend and change with the times, we must let go. Letting go is the most difficult thing we ever have to do, and an important part of letting go is learning how to forget.

To learn to forget one has to dispense with all excess baggage. Forgetting is letting things take their proper place; forgetting is learning how to abandon the small voice with the ready-made instructions; forgetting is knowing that something new lies ahead; forgetting is moving, flowing.

The ability to resign, to let go of obsolete responses, of exhausted relationships and of tasks beyond one's potential, is an essential part of the wisdom of living.
—FRITZ PERLS

86 Art experience

What happens when you perceive a work of art?

While nature provides us with plenty of profound esthetic experiences, the fine arts is where man-made beauty can allow us to experience altered states. What happens when we perceive a work of art? What combination of brain, mind, and body integrates what we are seeing or hearing into its own creative experience?

Our sensory organs play dominant and important roles. Our ears listen to vibrations and perceive harmonies, melodies, and rhythms. Our eyes feast on forms and visual representations that fill us with passion, fear, inspiration and so much more. Art's power, in its interactions with us and our integrations of the arts into our experience, are among the most stimulating, often pleasing and expansive experiences of our lives. A recent study found that encounters with perceptual vastness (in nature or in art) prompt a feeling of time dilation and awe and a transcending of self.

Eric R. Kandel, a Nobel Prize–winning neuroscientist and author, has probed and plumbed these extraordinary states of art experience and used science and history to weave a fascinating tour of what happens to us when we experience works of art. The summation of his scholarship and insight can be found in his book *The Age of Insight—The Quest to Understand the Unconscious in Art, Mind and Brain, from Vienna 1900 to the Present.*

Blending works as far ranging as the writings of Freud, the novels of Arthur Schnitzler, and the paintings of Gustav Klimpt, Oskar Kokoshka, and Egon Schiele, Kandel attempts to bridge art and science, often seen as being in conflict, in order to present a more complete picture of how minds and brains creatively respond to works of art. Kandel attempts to identify the areas of the brain where creative insights and appreciation occur. Early research points to the cerebral cortex's right hemisphere.

The next time you view a piece of art, consider how it is affecting your brain, your senses, your self.

Further Resources

Kandel's opus: *The Age of Insight—The Quest to Understand the Unconscious in Art, Mind and Brain, from Vienna 1900 to the Present,* runs to more than six hundred pages and contains hundreds of illustrations, some in color, as well as an extensive bibliography.

87 Creativity

Reach into yourself, find and make something new.

C reativity is something new, something fresh, something that arises out of the absence of preconceived ideas. Intuition—ideas that spring from the untapped, unpredictable parts of the self—results in creativity. To observe the unexpected, the unknown, and then use what one finds there in a new, unique way: That is creativity.

The process of creativity is an experience of ongoing attitudes, shifts, and changes that shape our way of relating to our environment. A great part of this process is perspective. When one has perspective, one has a good overview of a situation or an event; one can see clearly the emerging patterns in their various manifestations and configurations. With this perspective comes the ability to let the whole being consider a situation without hindrance and operate within the situation without premature conceptions.

Creativity is the ability to bring *something* into existence from *nothing*. That is, from chaos comes a meaningful, organized whole.

Further Resources

R esources on tapping into your creativity abound. Julia Cameron's classic *The Artist's Way* was rereleased as in a twentieth-anniversary edition in 2016. See also *Wired to Create* by Scott Barry Kaufman and Carolyn Gregoire; *Steal Like an Artist* by Austin Kleon; and *Creativity, Inc.* by Ed Catmull.

88 Profound esthetic experience

The high of contemplating beauty.

E sthetics is the branch of philosophy that deals with what is beautiful. Most often we think of it in relation to the fine arts. For many, "profound esthetic experience" sounds far away and generally inaccessible. But not so.

The model of the beautiful is nature, whether it be the world around us or the world within. Looking at a natural landscape can evoke a profound esthetic experience. So can focusing on a colorful, truly magnificent phosphene. What counts is awareness and openness.

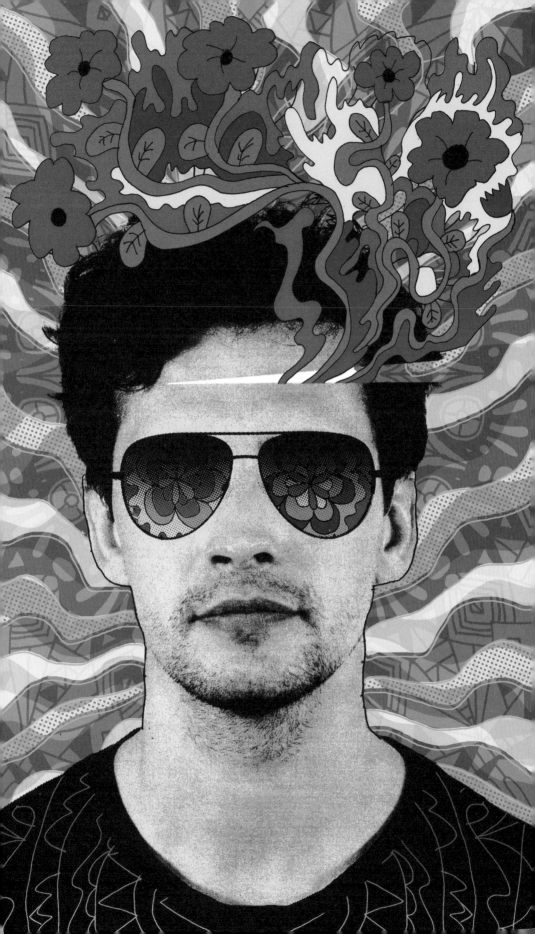

Further Resources

E. A. Gombrich's *Art and Illusion,* as well as the works of Bernard Berenson and Rudolf Arnheim, provide good material for consideration and instruction.

· ·

89 Flow

Being in the zone.

Psychologist Mihály Csíkszentmihályi describes the notion of "flow" as the psychology of optimal experience, "summarizing decades of research on the positive aspects of human experience—joy, creativity, the process of total involvement with life I call *flow.*" People in a full spectrum of life's domains have had the flow experience, from athletes who call their play "being in the zone," to writers who have felt as though their words are flowing through them without their complete knowledge.

Capturing the often elusive joy of life exemplified by the experience of flow cannot be achieved by any formulaic set of flow recipes. Instead, what Csíkszentmihályi does is to outline the general principles that can lead to a flow state. The focus on flow encompasses what Csíkszentmihályi calls the *autotelic* experience (from the Greek, *auto* represents self and *telos* represents the notion of having goals). An autotelic experience is one done for its own sake. An example cited is the surgeon who so enjoys the experience of his or her work that they would do it even without pay. Csíkszentmihályi found that when we engage in an activity that gives us both pleasure and an adequate challenge, we experience a state of ecstasy, and a sense of being separated from the cares and concerns of the everyday. In his opinion, to achieve a flow state, one must:

1 Be completely *focused.*

2 Feel a sense of *serenity.*

3 Feel a sense of *timelessness.*

4 Feel an inner *clarity.*

To create harmony in whatever one does is the last task that the flow theory presents to those who wish to attain optimal experience; it is a task that involves transforming the entirety of life into a single flow activity, with unified goals that provide constant purpose.
—MIHLÁY CSÍKSZENTMIHÁLYI

Find your favorite leisure activity that also challenges you, set your goal, focus, and your flow will find you. Your task should not be so challenging that it prompts anxiety and it shouldn't be so easy that it prompts boredom. Some common activities that create flow:

Writing

Improvising (comedy, rap, instrument-playing)

Painting

Playing a challenging game

Drawing

Intense teamwork (in sports, military training, etc.)

Further Resources

Csíkszentmihályi has written many books on flow, including *Flow: the Psychology of Optimal Experience*; *Finding Flow*; *Creativity*; *Flow in Sports* (with Susan A. Jackson); *Flow and the Foundations of Positive Psychology*; and *Applications of Flow in Human Development and Education*. Steven Kotler and Jamie Wheal's *Stealing Fire* discusses how Navy SEALs experience "group flow" in which their collective awareness, or "hive mind," makes them incredibly effective.

· ·

90 Peak experience

Giving birth, making love, and other activities that lead to deeper understanding.

Peak experiences are those highlights of our lives that give us awareness and insight into a deeper level of existence.

The peak experience is the event that changes our way of viewing reality. Peak experiences are similar to the transcendent awareness described by mystics and others who have undergone religious experiences. What makes the peak experience unique and different from the mystic and/or religious experience is its secular, naturalistic nature.

Peak experiences do not require the presence of the supernatural. They are characterized by the spontaneous awareness of some or all of the following points:

unity	time/space disorientation
nonjudgmental perception	receptivity
detachment and objectivity	transcendence of dichotomies
ego-transcendence	strong self-identity
self-trust	strong sense of "free will"
ends rather than means	humility and surrender

Peak experiences often occur during such diverse activities as making love, climbing a mountain, experiencing or creating a work of art, sailing, giving birth, reading, looking at a landscape, and listening.

For some people, peak experiences can remain in the memory as a reference point, making further peak experiences more accessible.

Further Resources

The works of Abe Maslow are reviewed in the resources of No. 118. Paul Bindrim's article "Facilitating Peak Experiences" appears in Otto and Mann's *Ways of Growth* and describes methods for realizing peak experiences. The discussion of the points frequently experienced with peak experiences is from Appendix A of Maslow's *Religions, Values, and Peak-Experiences*.

• •

91 Movement

Stay still. Burst forth! Feel the ways your body moves.

Although we may imagine "being at peace" in terms of stillness and serenity, the only constant is change.

Change is movement: being in action. To move is to be. Movement is our expression. Even when we are apparently still, we move; our insides pump and churn and strain and process.

Awareness of movement can come about through the absence of movement, through stillness. Feel the desire to push, to pull, to initiate. Know how to start, but be still. Move inside and feel movement inwardly before you do it.

Now move! Burst forth! Go out, be the world. But know what you move, how you move.

A good exercise is to move every part of the body, both as isolated parts and together with other parts; all sorts of ways you haven't tried before. Move your scalp, ears, eyes, lids, forehead, cheeks, jaw, neck, shoulders, back, spine, abdomen, arms, wrists, hands, fingers, elbows, pelvis, hips, thighs, knees, ankles, feet, and toes.

Move slowly, softly, sweetly, seriously, madly, happily, fleetingly; all of the ways you are.

92 Postures

Getting high with a handstand.

Stop reading and go and stand on your head for five minutes or do a shoulder stand. This is an excellent way to get high.

Postures are body gestures, positions sometimes natural, sometimes contrived, into which we can arrange our bodies. Postures help us to become our bodies, to become our selves.

Postures, body positions, and physical actions that bring about awareness include:

stretching

holding

twisting

expanding

contracting

knotting (intertwining the limbs)

sitting

standing

lying

crouching

touching

turning

hunkering (a crouch with the buttocks as near to the floor as possible)

raising the limbs

pushing

pulling

tapping

lifting

slapping

shaking

93 Tensing

Feel your muscles relax and awaken.

Relax. That's the first thing to do when tensing. Tensing is the deliberate, conscious play of the musculature. There are many methods that will teach you how to relax; what is fundamental is to learn how you *don't* relax.

You can try it now by sitting down in a chair with your back straight. Put your right hand on the back of your neck so that you can feel the different muscles there. Relax. While still touching and feeling your neck with your hand slowly raise your left leg off the ground, bring your knee as close to the chest as possible, without altering your position.

Could you feel the muscles in your neck tense and shift as you raised your leg? Could you experience how you use muscles that are not directly connected with the action you are carrying out?

While still sitting, totally relax as much as possible. Now deliberately tense the muscles in your right forearm by making a very tight fist. Continue to increase the tension until your arm begins to quiver and shake. Then relax. Repeat this process two more times until you can experience the dynamics of your tension/relaxation cycles. Try the same procedure with other sets of muscles.

Further Resources

Edmund Jacobson's *Progressive Relaxation* is a classic and is still an authoritative text in this area. Also see Bernard Gunther's *Sense Relaxation.*

94 Jumping up and down

Higher, higher, higher . . .

I am not really qualified to talk about this method. Only certain masters know its full potential. When wrongfully employed, JUAD (Jumping Up And Down) can bring about severe mental aberration and radical psychic transformations.

To begin with, you should be standing. It is much better to practice JUAD out of doors, on grass, where, if you fall, you will not be seriously injured.

Ball both hands up into fists, and keep your hands this way throughout the JUAD. Then begin to crouch down, bending the torso and the knees. Some find that it helps to bend the arms at the elbows. When you are almost in a full crouch, use the power of your legs to propel your body upward. The aim is to actually leave the ground and soar high into the air. Try to land flat on your feet. Don't stop. Repeat the above procedure, trying to go higher and higher each time.

Keep going higher. If JUAD is done properly, you'll never come down. If a real JUAD master is required, find one who is under eight years old.

· ·

95 Play

Games allow us to explore new ways of being.

"Tag: you're it," you exclaim as you run from the room. Going through doors, room to room, she'll never find you here. Quick, behind the curtains, she's already in the next room. That was too close. Should you still hide or move while you can, while there's still time?

We all have played and some of us continue to play. In the beginning of our lives we play spontaneously, with ourselves, with others, with objects, even with figments of our imagination. As we age and grow into adults, our childish notions of play are curtailed and we reserve play for things like sports, drama, and games. More recently, with the rise of computer and video games, more and more adults are spending more time playing than grownups did in the past.

How do these new playtimes affect adults? Are they making us happier? Calmer? Yes, play often does. There are many benefits to play, both psychological and physical.

- Physical sensations abound: adrenaline flows, breathing is altered, and heart rates change as our blood flows through our bodies.

- Play is fantasy made manifest, with unfettered imagination spontaneously summoned into action.

- Games are safe spaces to explore new ways of being, to take risks, to be adventurous, to explore new dynamics with our peers.

In 1938, Johan Huizinga, a cultural theorist and historian from the Netherlands, wrote a groundbreaking book, *Homo Ludens—The Play Element of Culture*, with a new theory of the nature of play in the development of culture and, as a result, society. Huizinga views play as a major basis of human experience. The book's title is a play on Homo sapiens (roughly: "wise man") and Homo faber ("man the maker"); instead, with "ludens," Huizinga posits man as a player. While the personal benefits of play are important, Huizinga also notes its essential role in society: "Civilization is, in its earliest phases, played. It does not come from play like a baby detaching itself from the womb: it arises in and as play, and never leaves it."

Huizinga defines some five aspects that characterize play: play is free; play is not like "real life"—it is nonordinary; play is different from ordinary life in location and in duration; play creates its own order; play is not-for-profit, i.e., it has no "material" interest.

Homo Ludens has inspired many theorists and philosophers and is at the root of contemporary game theory. What's more, with automation now threatening more and more jobs, and the definition of work being reworked continuously, play becomes a much more important aspect of our future lives.

Go play: Go outside, jump rope, jump up and down, play tag, play hide and seek, play with life's mysteries. Don't think, be like a child. Be like an adult: Stay inside, play a game, go online, play with others. To all: Be players, at any time, be *homo ludens*.

Further Resources

Homo Ludens—The Play Element of Culture by Johan Huizinga.

• •

96 Running
Nothing beats a runner's high.

Running is a fine way to alter consciousness. It is accessible and can be great fun. However, before beginning serious running or any other vigorous exercises, it is advisable to get a checkup from a doctor.

When you start running, begin slowly; build up your confidence, endurance, ability, and speed and eventually you will be able to run distances you never imagined. Running gets you high in the same way as many other techniques offered here: by altering your breathing. When you run, you change your breathing and the amount of oxygen reaching your brain. This in turn alters consciousness. Running also changes the speed of your heart and this, too, can alter consciousness.

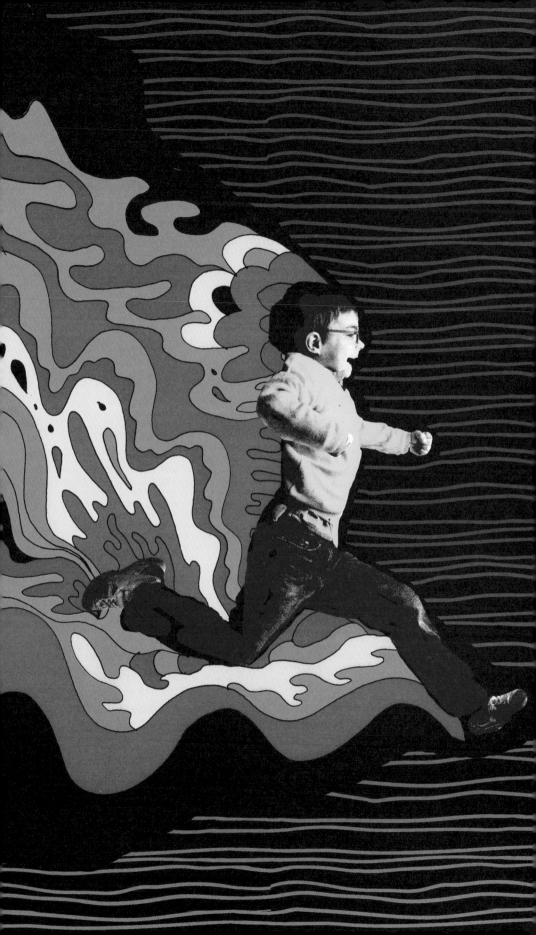

The difference between running and jogging is speed. When you jog, you move along at what might be the equivalent of a horse's trot. When you run, you're cantering. When you sprint, you're into your own version of the gallop. Running and sprinting cause your heart to beat much faster than normal, jogging does not. The long-distance runners in the Andes Mountains in South America have been tested and shown to have a slower than average heartbeat and pulse. This is because when they are running their hearts speed up, but after they have stopped running their hearts slow down to a level lower than before they had begun running. This is not true for someone who runs once a month or even once a week, but applies only to those who run every day.

Real running requires both effort and practice. If you are going to run a mile, you should do so in under eight minutes. You can run five miles at a somewhat slower pace and achieve the same results: an altered state of consciousness.

Further Resources

Dr. Tim Noakes's *Lore of Running* gives detailed information on how fast to run, for how long, and what running will do to your heart and circulatory system. For philosophical takes on the sport, see George Sheehan's classic *Running and Being* and novelist Haruki Murakami's memoir, *What I Talk About When I Talk About Running.* No running library would be complete without Christopher McDougall's *Born to Run: A Hidden Tribe, Superathletes, and the Greatest Race the World Has Never Seen,* which offers a fascinating look into the practices of the Tarahumara Indians, ultramarathoners in Mexico.

· ·

97 Gymnastics
Unleash your body's potential.

Doing somersaults, handsprings, and various flips and dives can alter consciousness. Working out with rings, parallel bars, the pommel horse, and rope will do the same thing, and allow you to develop personal coordination and grace. These need to be done properly so that you do not injure yourself.

Gymnastics are similar to running in that they really make your heart and your lungs work hard.

98 Golf

Simple sport or spiritual journey?

Ecstatic experience and adventure lurk in the queerest of places. Michael Murphy, founder of the Esalen Institute, stopped off in Scotland many years ago on his way to India. While in Scotland he played some golf and had, as a result, some of the richest mystical experiences of his life.

Murphy's mythical master of golf, Shivas Irons, initiated him into a system where golf symbolizes the true spiritual potentialities of the human soul. Golf is seen as the transcendental journey, not so much as a venture to get somewhere as a mythical circumnavigation of inner space. The components of the journey, those that lead to spiritual reunification, include a study of the whiteness of the ball, the mystery of the golf cup and the cup as a metaphor for the doorways in ordinary life, the art of replacing the divot, and the study of true gravity as produced by the backswing.

Speaking of Shivas Irons's ideal, Murphy concludes:

> His ideal would have us know his Body and this Dance, would have us live in it while playing golf and singing ballads and talking to our friends; yes, and even while we are trying to pass it on to others.

Further Resources

Michael Murphy has described his experiences of and thoughts on golf in his novel *Golf in the Kingdom*. Also see Arnold Haultain's 1908 classic, *The Mystery of Golf*, and articles and books by golfer Bob Toski.

99 Mountaineering and rock climbing

Where breath, awareness, and beauty combine.

Whether you have sought out a local mountain or are climbing in the Himalayas with full pack, gear, special equipment, and Sherpa guides, mountaineering can be a fantastic adventure. It requires not only physical endurance and fortitude but also skill, and keen attention and awareness.

What makes mountaineering a means to alter consciousness is a combination of factors. First there are the surroundings. The natural elevation of mountain summits over the surrounding land affords the climber magnificent views and vistas, as well as new environmental perspectives. By climbing high, you are also changing the oxygen composition of the air you are breathing. The higher above sea level you are, the less oxygen there is in the air you breathe. The effort required to climb most mountains and rock faces will change your breathing pattern and your heartbeat. These in turn will change the amount of oxygen reaching your brain and make you high.

Another factor affecting mountaineers is the negatively ionized air high above sea level. Most urban environments abound in positively ionized air. (See No. 230.)

By climbing mountains you are facing a challenge. Successful completion of the challenge, the endurance of hardships along the way, and the exercise of your skills can provide unique sensations. The trip down can be equally exciting and exhilarating.

Further Resources

Mountaineering: Freedom of the Hills, considered the bible of climbing by many mountaineers, is now in its ninth edition; it includes a bibliography and a list of films. The mountain climb as a metaphor for the metaphysical quest is presented in René Daumal's Mount Analogue, which was made into a movie called The Holy Mountain by Alexandro Jodorowsky.

100 Mushroom hunting

The forest has much to reveal.

World-renowned photographer Frank Spinelli shared his love of foraging for mushrooms in the forest and what special kinds of altered states of consciousness it creates. You're in a place of nature and you're looking for treasure.

As a treasure hunter in the forest, you can experience a new kind of calm, in quiet, peaceful surroundings. There's the nativistic feelings of sensations as you explore a new environment and the many new species that surround you as you forage. You're out of your element, surrounded by nature; you're inside a living organism and in a brand new realm. Each new part of the forest has much to reveal to you.

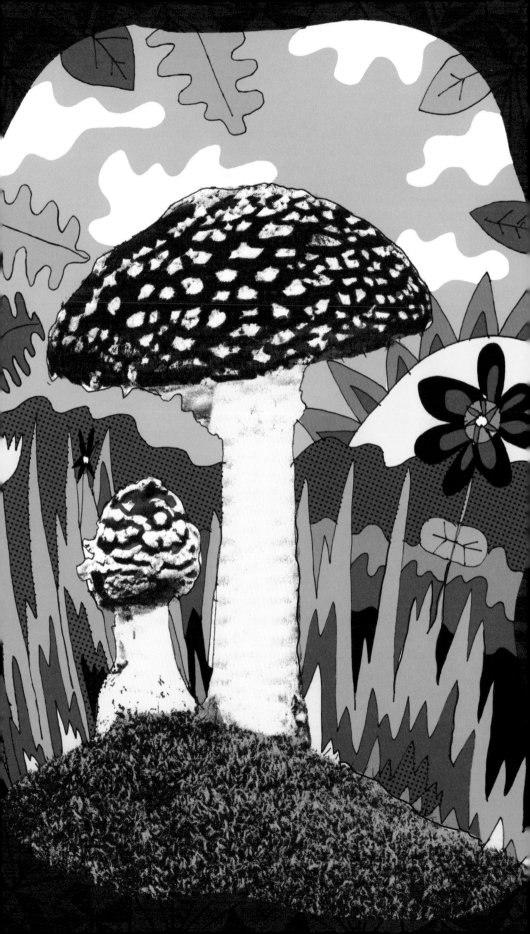

The mushrooms, the object of your endeavor, may or may not be there. Or they may be in another location, for another day. And if you find mushrooms to eat, there's the intense satisfaction of having searched for and discovered food; this is very different than buying food in a store or a restaurant. You've done it yourself; you found it.

The mushroom hunt brings the hunter back to an earlier version of humankind. As you walk through the forest looking for mushrooms, you can sense the roots of being a hunter-gatherer, making contact with a primordial state of being. You can experience the wonder of finding what you're looking for, finding mushrooms, food you can eat, and even more. Looking for mushrooms in the forest can be very transcendental.

Further Resources

Frank says he usually reserves his mushroom finds to the nine mushroom species that he knows from his long foraging experiences are not poisonous. He said that most anyone can use the internet to identify five or six mushroom types that are safe to eat. Another expansive view of the nature of fungus can be found in the extensive work of mycologist Paul Stamets (fungi.com).

· ·

101 Survival tests

Push your body and mind to new heights.

Many cultures once used survival tests to initiate young boys into the adult life of the community. The survival test allowed the boy to act as an adult for the first time, to prove himself to his fellow men, and to show what he had learned from his upbringing in the community.

Contemporary versions of the survival test exist in the U.S. military, especially in the Rangers and in civilian groups like Outward Bound. The Rangers and other branches of the services have been known to test graduates of their training by parachuting them into desert, jungle, or forest areas, miles from civilization, with only their parachutes and the clothes on their back. Most of the participants make it back to civilization and some report altered consciousness as a result of lack of food, intensity of effort, isolation, and exhilaration.

Further Resources

Outward Bound lists its trips on its website (outwardbound.org). There are wilderness survival schools across the country. Check your local listings for a program near you.

· ·

102 Futures

Life can only be understood backwards;
but it must be lived forwards.

—SØREN KIERKEGAARD, PHILOSOPHER

Future consciousness, which, needless to say, is an altered state of consciousness, is no longer a game or occupation; it is now a necessity. The future is too close at hand to ignore. Its seeming presence encourages thoughtfulness and serious considerations. We live in a time of often exponential changes. Science and technology alter our lives seemingly every week. In addition, the flow of life into cities worldwide and the almost daily changes in climate, no matter how they occur, combine to make our always-on style of life ever more challenging and full of momentous alterations and transformations. If we don't think about, plan, and act to make our future better now, when will we have the time to do so? Now, or never?

The future of the past is in the future

The future of the present is in the past

The future of the future is in the present
—JOHN MCHALE, ARTIST, SOCIOLOGIST, AND SPECIALIST IN FUTURE STUDIES

I am vitally interested in the future. After all, I'll be spending the rest of my life there.
—CHARLES KETTERING, WORLD FUTURE SOCIETY

Further Resources

There are several hundred new books and articles dealing with the future every year. Three good texts to begin an inquiry would be John McHale's *The Future of the Future,* Arthur C. Clarke's *Profiles of the Future,* and M. J. Dunstan and P. W. Garlan's *Worlds in the Making. The Futurist* was a bimonthly periodical that covered the whole field. It ceased publication in 2015, but its publisher, the World Future Society, still makes back issues available. The best current source for articles and videos concerning future trends is from the website Reddit (reddit.com/r/futurology).

. . . .

103 Acceleration and future shock

Adjusting to rapid changes.

"Future shock," as defined for us by Alvin Toffler in his seminal book of the same name, is very much like the culture shock one encounters when traveling. Suddenly you're out of your familiar environment, out of your type of society. All the cues you once used to judge right from wrong, good from bad, no longer fit. In the new culture, the old way of doing things won't do. The effects are dizzying, and often it's a relief to get home, to get back to the familiar, to know what works.

Future shock describes the effect of rapid change hurtling us faster and faster into a future world. Nothing lasts: rules, regulation, cultural cues; they're all falling by the wayside as we go, full speed, into our future. What worked yesterday can barely get us by today and will be totally inadequate tomorrow.

And there is no home to go back to; the retreat, through nostalgia, to a more familiar past, just makes life more difficult.

More recently, futurists like Ray Kurzweil have documented and called attention to the accelerations taking place in many areas of contemporary technology and other aspects of planetary society and culture. Everything is speeding up.

Perhaps the most incredible example of this acceleration is what's known as Moore's Law. Gordon Moore, then an executive at chip-making company Fairchild Semiconductor (a precursor of Intel) published an article in the journal *Electronics* in 1965 predicting that every eighteen to twenty-four months, the number of components that could be fit on a computer chip would double, yet the price of a chip would remain relatively constant. He had no idea how right he would be.

As a result of the success of Moore's Law for more than half a century (!!), we now can have what used to be referred to as a supercomputer in our mobile phones.

Further Resources

Alvin Toffler's *Future Shock* has many references to follow up for further investigation. See also Kurzweil's "Law of Accelerating Returns" and his books *The Age of Spiritual Machines* and *The Singularity Is Near: When Humans Transcend Biology.*

....

104 Voluntary social withdrawal

Transcend society by pulling away from it.

Often it becomes necessary, after one has spent a long time seeking essential and personal universals, to enter into a new phase where insights and epiphanies resulting from alterations of consciousness are allowed to coalesce. This integrative process can often be furthered in an isolated situation. The length of time spent in voluntary social withdrawal must vary according to the individual and need not be a full retreat from social spheres. It may be an afternoon alone in an apartment, a walk alone in the woods, or two years alone on an island.

There is the danger that social withdrawal will prove seductively attractive, and one will be tempted to drop out permanently. When this happens it is usually because illusion has superseded the sense of reality. Dropping out can be used creatively to assimilate new data about one's culture, but staying dropped out usually means lapsing into rationalizations, believing that one is superior to society at large.

Voluntary social withdrawal allows a new phase of aware consciousness to develop. When this temporary withdrawal is combined with cultural assimilation (see No. 12), and the individual is able to maintain the insights and universals of previous altered states of consciousness and develop the ability to transcend cultural patterns, then the final stage of maturational integration begins: The individual is involved in and awakened by what happens every day (see No. 106).

....

105 Communes

A different way of living and bonding.

Concomitant with mass alterations of middle-class consciousness in the 1960s countercultural revolution, by way of drug usage, new sexual expression, and future shock, came the first beginnings of an attempt to retribalize society by communes. Communes afforded an opportunity for those who wanted to experiment with different lifestyles to gather together and put their theories into practice. Some have tried not having any theories at all and have been founded on the rule of no rules.

This came about, in part, when certain groups found that altering consciousness by way of drugs and other methods required new ways of living together. Some felt that the old structures, like stable homes and family situations, no longer fit their experiences of reality. They needed to retreat from society in order to test the social implications of their experiences and new modes of consciousness and awareness. Communal living seemed to provide a safe way to try out new ways of being and at the same time served as a statement against social forms that many communards felt were the manifestations of a highly structured, linear, bureaucratic culture. They felt that their communes were a sign of life in a dying society.

By being forced to live closely on a day-to-day basis with people outside their immediate families, members had the opportunity to experiment with different ways of experiencing reality. Many communes have failed, some due to idealism, others due to economics or poor organization; but some continue.

Further Resources

A fine Canadian periodical in this field, *Alternate Society,* ceased publication in 2014 but is still available on microform (catalogue.nla.gov.au). The Fellowship for International Community contains a webpage devoted to resources concerning communes (ic.org).

• •

106 Everyday experience

The joy of just being.

If the doors of perception were cleansed every thing would appear to man as it is, infinite.
—WILLIAM BLAKE

The "supreme reason" does not lie in the domain of mystical visions of any kind.
—SUZUKI DAISETZ, BUDDHIST AUTHOR

A monk asked Ummon, "What is the Buddha?" "It is a shit-wiping stick," replied Ummon.
—CASE XXI OF THE MUMONKAN

Joshu asked Nansen, "What is the Way?" Nansen answered, "Your ordinary mind—that is the Way." Joshu said, "Does it go in any particular direction?" Nansen replied, "The more you seek after it, the more it runs away." Joshu: "Then how can you know it is the Way?" Nansen: "The Way does not belong to knowing or not knowing. Knowing is illusion. Not knowing is lack of discrimination. When you get to this unperplexed Way, it is like the vastness of space, an unfathomable void, so how can it be this or that, yes or no?" Upon this Joshu came to a sudden realization.
—CASE XIX OF THE MUMONKAN

"I do not ask you about last month, or about next month. I ask you to say something about here and now." None of the monks responded to this, so Ummon said, "Every Day is a good Day."
—CASE VI OF THE HEKIGANROKU

A monk asked, "What is my own self?"

"Have you finished your rice gruel (breakfast?)" asked the Master (Joshu).

"Yes, I have finished it," replied the monk.

"Then go and wash your dishes," said the Master.
—FROM THE TRANSMISSION OF THE LAMP, CHUAN 10

If you understand, things are such as they are;

If you do not understand, things are such as they are—
—GENSHA

Before enlightenment, chop wood, carry water;

After enlightenment, chop wood, carry water.
—ZEN DUST

This is it. There's nothing hidden at all. Nothing special. *Tada* (*only* this, *just* this, nothing but). The final alteration of consciousness is the perception of things as they are. To perceive the world without excess, without fetters. To be in the moment.

When you eat, *just* eat. When you sleep, *just* sleep. You are: *just* be.

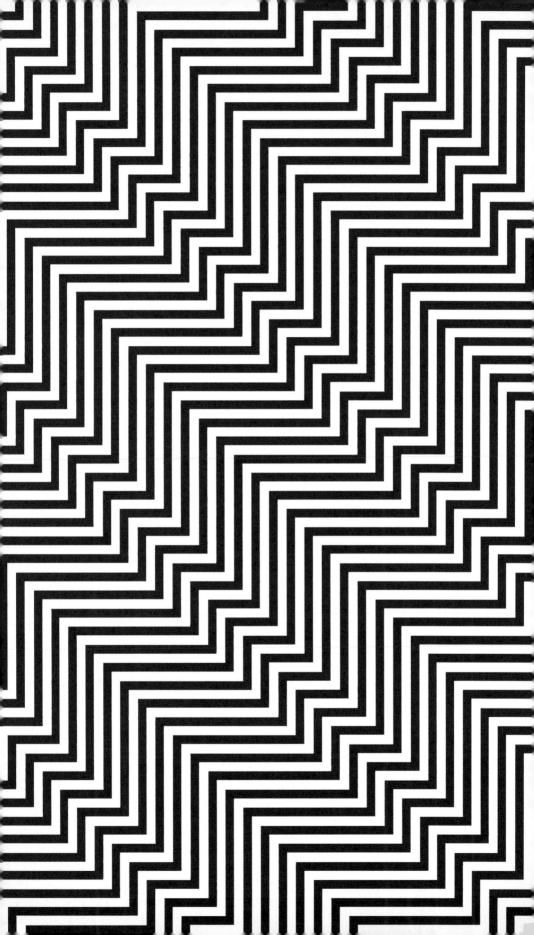

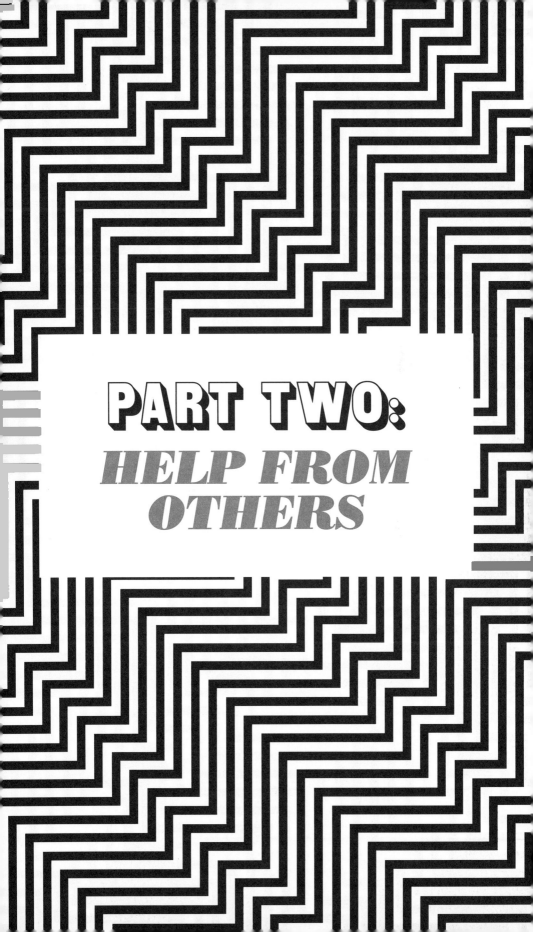

PART TWO:
HELP FROM OTHERS

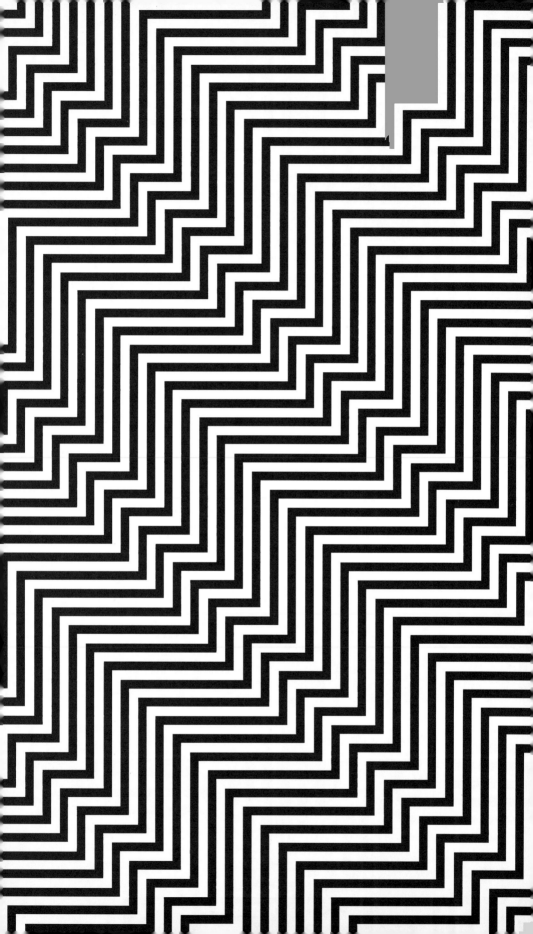

CHAPTER 6

THERAPIES AND MISCELLANEOUS

I n this section are included brief descriptions of a number of psychotherapies. Chosen are those psychotherapeutic techniques that attempt to change or alter the individual's perception of themselves and their world. The methods covered are those which have proved especially successful, either as models or schools of thought assimilated by the culture. When psychotherapy is successful, it effects an altered state of consciousness.

107 Psychoanalysis

Uncover your unconscious.

S igmund Freud, as is well known, developed a system of therapy aimed at the cure of mental and nervous disorders; it is known as psychoanalysis. Only the bare bones are presented here. There is more literature on psychoanalysis than on any other form of psychotherapy.

Freud developed his system working with Josef Breuer on the treatment of hysterics through hypnotic techniques. If hypnosis could cure physical ailments, Freud thought, the root cause of certain ailments must have been mental. After some experimentation, Freud began to formulate general theories of the structure of the mind and therapies based on these theories.

He described the mind as divided into the *unconscious* (the seat of repressed material) and the *conscious* (the part that is in contact with the environment).

The unconscious is ruled by the *id*, the original animal-like portion of the mind or self, which also houses the *libido*, which he characterized as being primarily sexual in nature. Out of the id develops the *ego*, which attempts to deal with the external world while still helping to satisfy the

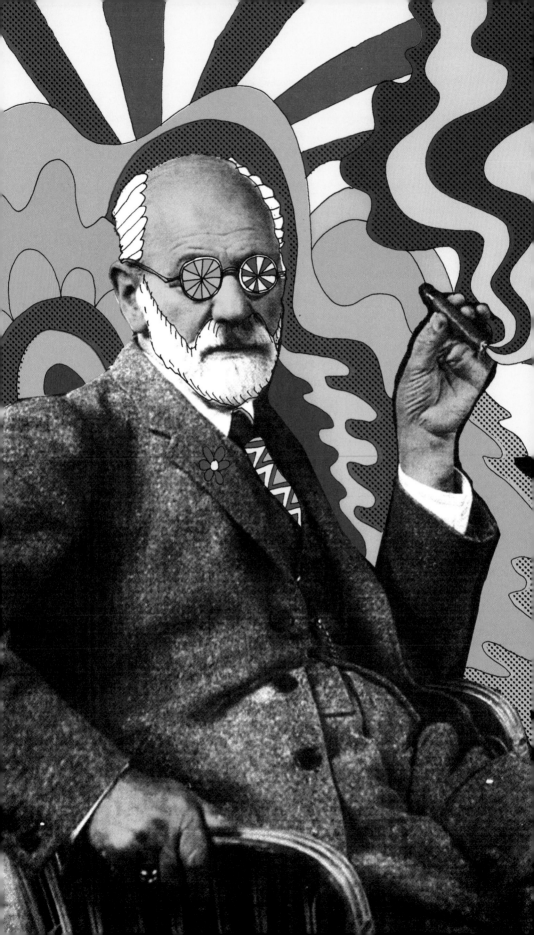

baser needs and drives of the id. But the ego is also serving a second master, the conscience, which Freud referred to as the *superego*. It is the superego that internalizes parental prohibitions. The superego is a perfectionist.

Generally, the patient in psychoanalysis says whatever enters their mind while lying on a couch from which they cannot see the analyst (the psychoanalytic practitioner) sitting behind them, listening, and taking notes. The talking is linked to Freud's theories of catharsis: by verbally expressing the nature and source of their problems, the patient will be able to recontact repressed feelings and drives. Some of this newly contacted energy becomes available for healthy living. The patient expresses whatever comes to mind, letting associations come freely and allowing the repressed material to guide their talking.

Another important aspect of psychoanalysis is the theory of transference. Transference occurs when the patient transfers strong emotional feeling, such as love and hate, from the person they actually love or hate to the psychoanalyst. The importance of transference is that it gives the patient an opportunity to solve many problems by proxy—that is, by allowing the analyst to emotionally "stand in" for the real object of love or hate.

Freud pictured man as being highly complex: as living in reality and operating under rational principles and yet also living in fantasies and dreams, operating under conflict and confusion. The mature individual can cope with these inconsistencies and ambivalences. His very complexity is one major root of his maturity.

Freud had many disciples who went on to form their own schools of psychological thought. Wilhelm Reich, Otto Rank, and Carl Jung, among others, will be considered separately. Alfred Adler, another follower, believed that Freud did not deal properly with the importance of feelings of inferiority. He also placed high value on the social relationship between the therapist and the patient. This is also evident in the interpersonal theories of personality developed by Harry Stack Sullivan. Erik Erikson brings much social behavior to bear on psychoanalytic theory. Both Adler and Wilhelm Stekel believed that Freud emphasized the past too heavily in psychoanalysis.

Further Resources

The Modern Library edition of *The Basic Writings of Sigmund Freud* coupled with Ernest Jones's *The Life and Work of Sigmund Freud* will provide a good introduction to the field of psychoanalysis.

. . . .

108 Analytical psychology
Tapping into a universal unconscious.

C arl Gustav Jung is easily the most extraordinary scholarly talent to emerge from the psychoanalytic group. Though the basis of his psychological theories and practice centered around analytical psychology, Jung's interests ranged literally from alchemy to Zen Buddhism.

Many believe that his most important role in contemporary psychology was his interest in and acceptance of Eastern ways of thought and wisdom. His basically open intellectual stance allowed him to draw material from a variety of sources. He was thereby in a position to integrate the psycho-philosophical truths expressed in Eastern religio-psycho-philosophical systems into his decidedly Western *Weltanschauung* (German for "world view").

After breaking with Freud, Jung went on to build a system of psychology based on a desexualized libido. In addition, Jung sought to interpret behavior rather than discover its causes. He believed (as Freud did) that there was a *personal unconscious,* which contained our own repressed memories, but also that there was a *collective unconscious,* which contained our repressed awareness of everything that has ever happened. Jung felt that he had observed the existence of certain *archetypes,* or universal associations, that stemmed from the creative forces of this collective unconscious shared and tapped by all mankind. The collective unconscious is not the same as an individual's unconscious. Rather, it contains so much of humankind's conscious and unconscious: memories, ancestral strands woven into all of our DNA, and the sum of all experiences. To contemplate and reflect upon the nature of this collective unconscious gives access to our birthrights, our instincts, and our shared experiences as well as our collective destinies.

The nature of the psychotherapeutic practice of analytical psychology seeks to explore and understand the individual's relationship to the collective unconscious. In addition to this shared unconscious, Jung divided personality into *persona,* the social mask, and *ego,* the conscious and unconscious parts of the personality responsible for personal behavior.

Throughout his works, one sees the influence of and interest in a variety of areas including the study of the phenomena of the self, the development of culture, flying saucers, Taoist yoga, Tibetan Buddhism, religion and spiritual needs, dreams, symbols, Taoist and Western alchemy, Zen, art, and literature.

Further Resources

Jung's collected works have been published in eighteen volumes by the Bollingen Foundation. His autobiography, *Memories, Dreams, Reflections*, is both enlightening and entertaining. Selections of his thought have been edited by his associate Jolande Jacobi under the title *Psychological Reflections. Man and His Symbols,* a volume of papers edited by Jung and beautifully designed by Aldus Books in London, may be the best introduction to Jung's ideas.

109 Character analysis

A body-oriented approach to therapy.

Of all the theoretical developments of Wilhelm Reich, his work on character analysis and body psychotherapy have had the most profound influence on therapeutic interventions.

A psychoanalyst by training, Reich's real importance came with the attention that he paid to the body of the patient. He was the first of the psychoanalytic school to pay attention to the patient's posture, especially as an expression of personal character. Reich felt that the patient's physical stance—which he dubbed "character armor"—unconsciously expressed defenses against the analytic process (and, subsequently, defense against the unveiling of his unconscious processes). He would make the patient aware of these defenses and the resultant character armor, typically expressed in muscle tension and rigidity, and he would analyze the sources of the resistant character formation.

Though most classical analysts respect his work on character, it is only in recent years that Reich's work as a whole has come under serious consideration, especially by those practicing body-oriented approaches to psychotherapy.

Further Resources

Character Analysis is the title of Reich's book on the description of his psychoanalytic method. A good introduction to his later work is to be found in *Wilhelm Reich: Selected Writings*, which includes a bibliography. Today, body psychotherapy is practiced in many forms across the world. See the United States Association for Body Psychotherapy (usabp.org) for educational resources and a directory of practitioners.

· ·

110 Psychodrama and drama therapy
Reaching new insights through performance.

P sychodrama is a system developed by J. L. Moreno as a technique used in group psychotherapy and has powerful and far-reaching applications.

Moreno points out that the word "drama" comes from the transliteration of a Greek word that really means "action" or "things done." He sees psychodrama as a technique for reaching the truth through dramatic means, by acting out one's feelings. Whereas drama therapy involves fictionalized scenes and theater exercises, psychodrama—a blend of group therapy and performance—specifically focuses on addressing an individual's problem by acting out a situation portraying an issue or conflict experienced by a participant. Moreno defines five necessary instruments for psychodrama.

1   The stage: a safe environment for psychological action.

2   The subject or actor: This is the man or woman who chooses to be on the stage to present his or her interior and personal world through the psychodramatic technique.

3   The director (usually the therapist): He or she fulfills three basic roles: the producer, the counselor, and the analyst. It is the responsibility of the director to be aware of clues from the subject and to turn those clues (to the subject's inner dynamics) into dramatic action. The director may attack the subject or support the subject, depending on what is necessary in the course of dramatic action.

4   The staff of auxiliary egos: These staff members have their function in playing out the other characters involved in the protagonist's world. They must serve his needs as well as supplement his acting and his behavior.

5   The audience: This group has a dual purpose. By presenting public opinion, the audience can attempt to help the subject. By being itself, it can gain help by observing what occurs on the stage. It is the responsibility of the director to guide the audience as well as the subject.

The process of bringing feelings to the surface through psychodrama can lead to new emotional insights. The performance not only allows the actor to see his situation from a new perspective, it also creates a safe space for exploring new relationship dynamics and solutions to problems. In recent years, as the practice of psychodrama has decreased, its influence on other therapeutic approaches has grown, especially drama therapy and Gestalt therapy (No. 117).

Further Resources

J. L. Moreno's work is explained in his book *Who Shall Survive?,* which includes a complete bibliography. *Psychodrama* provides specific details on the dramatic technique. The American Society of Group Psychotherapy and Psychodrama (asgpp.org) provides publications, events, and a directory of certified psychodramatists across the country.

• •

111 Logotherapy
Finding your meaning.

Logotherapy was developed by the existential analyst Viktor Frankl. The name is taken from the Greek *logo,* translated as "meaning and spirit."

When asked to give a one-sentence definition of logotherapy, Frankl replied: "In logotherapy the patient sits on a chair and hears things he finds unpleasant to hear."

Frankl contends that because man is the only animal who seeks meaning, because man is the only animal who worries, this meaning is the source of the very spirit of the human condition. In logotherapy he attempts to help the patient discover his own "will to meaning."

A logotherapist will lead the patient to what Frankl believes to be the major stumbling block in all human development: lack of meaning. When life has no purpose, the patient will be unable to function in a world where values have no connection with his own personality. The task of logotherapy is to help the patient experience for himself his own personal meaning of life.

Frankl derived a great many of his psychological insights from experiences he had in a German concentration camp during World War II. In the camp, Frankl regularly saw people die from lack of hope. He came to correlate positive, active consciousness with mental health and, conversely, mental passivity with mental illness. This mental passivity he saw was characterized by a feeling of nothingness, which he came to call the "existential vacuum." After leaving the camp and entering private practice, Frankl saw many patients exhibiting depressive symptoms that paralleled those that he had seen in the camp. Complaints detailed feelings of nothingness and lack of meaning in life. By confronting his patients with their emptiness and urging them to take personal responsibility for their condition, he was able to help patients develop and recognize strong meaning in life. This led to further ownership of will and, eventually, to health.

How does one find meaning? Frankl suggested several ways:

1   by creating a work or doing a deed

2   by experiencing something or encountering someone

3   by the attitude we take toward unavoidable suffering. As Frankl said, "When we are no longer able to change a situation . . . we are challenged to change ourselves."

Further Resources

Frankl's logotherapy is set forth and expanded upon in two of his works: *The Doctor and the Soul: From Psychotherapy to Logotherapy* and *Man's Search for Meaning.*

• •

112 Existential therapy

Accepting mortality leads to more authentic living.

Existential therapy is born out of existential philosophy. There are elements of Kierkegaard's emphasis on agency (the individual is responsible for giving meaning to life and living it authentically), Nietzsche's examination of meaninglessness, and even Ernest Becker's late twentieth-century study of death denial (the innate desire to transcend death via "immortality projects" like religion, creative pursuits, offspring, etc.).

One of the first examples of the blending of philosophy and therapy was *Daseinsanalyse,* an existential psychoanalytic system developed by Ludwig Binswanger and greatly influenced by the philosophy of Martin Heidegger. *Da* means "there"; *sein* means "being"; thus, *Daseinsanalyse* means, literally, "being there." It is often referred to as "being-in-the-world." The assumptions begin with "there" being taken as a *personal* "there." Because man can become aware of his "being-there" he can become responsible for his being. His being then goes from "being-in-itself" to an extension: "being-for-itself."

Contemporary therapists like Irvin Yalom apply these theories to a therapy based on the acceptance of ultimate truths (meaninglessness, isolation, death, freedom) to make better, more authentic decisions in the here and now.

Psychologist Rollo May took a more hopeful stance, stating that we all have a limitless potential to be any type of person and it is our responsibility to recognize that we have that potential. Often people choose to ignore their potential (pathologically) in an attempt to function in their environments, like a plant growing toward the light but falling over, and the therapy focuses on reminding the person that they can choose to act differently in the world than they are acting.

Further Resources

An overview of *Daseinsanalyse* is presented in Binswanger's *Being-In-The-World*. Rollo May's *Existence* covers other developments in existential psychology. Irvin Yalom has written many books, including fiction and stories (e.g., *When Nietzsche Wept, The Schopenhauer Cure,* and *The Spinoza Problem*) as well as nonfiction (e.g., *Existential Psychotherapy* and *The Gift of Therapy*).

· ·

113 Rational psychotherapy

Situations do not cause feelings; beliefs do.

Rational psychotherapy, also known as rational-emotive psychotherapy, holds that man's emotions are caused and controlled by thinking. It is the development of Albert Ellis, who held that someone experiencing positive emotions is reinforcing those feelings, influencing them with thoughts like "this is good." "This is bad" would tend to cause a negative emotional experience. These phrases are usually subvocal and often not part of awareness.

The aim of the therapy is to help the patient understand and realize what internalized sentences are now the basis of their thoughts. Once this is discovered, the patient is encouraged to substitute more positive, more rational, and more realistic supportive sentences. It is believed that this sentence substitution will help the patient to change their own behavior.

In this respect, rational psychotherapy is like many of the "positive-thinking" philosophies. Ellis encourages his patients to realize that they control their own destinies through the way they deal with problems and the way they talk to themselves.

Our patients . . . frequently remark: "I can't stand it when things go wrong.". . . we quickly interrupt: "What do you mean you can't stand *it*? *It* doesn't really exist—it is just a figment of your imagination. What you really mean to say is: "I can't stand myself when things go wrong—because I falsely tell myself that things shouldn't go wrong, or that I'm no good for letting them go wrong. But if I stopped telling myself this nonsense, then I could fairly easily stand—though never perhaps like—the frustrations of the world and could respect myself for being able to accept these frustrations."

Ellis's theories laid the groundwork for the cognitive behavioral therapy movement (see No. 127), which remains very popular today.

Further Resources

Ellis's initial statement of theory was presented in his book *How to Live with a "Neurotic" at Home and at Work*. Also consult *A Guide to Rational Living* and *Reason and Emotion in Psychotherapy* for later changes in viewpoint. The quote above is from *A Guide to Rational Living*.

• •

114 General semantics

How do symbols influence our thinking?

General semantics was recognized and formulated by Alfred Korzybski. Korzybski is best known for his work on words as symbols, their usage, and their meanings. Much of his work involved examinations of symbols and their relationships to the things that they symbolize. These studies led to his analysis of the influence of symbols on behavior.

Korzybski found that human beings have a unique property that arises from their manipulation of symbols: time-binding. Time-binding indicates the preservation of memories and the recording of experiences for the use of subsequent generations. This time-binding is usually accomplished through the use of language.

Language is a verbal map of a nonverbal territory. But language carries with it culturally acquired powers that influence the user of language to mistake the map for the territory it attempts to describe. This is similar to believing the name and advertising credo of Kool cigarettes is accurate even when confronted with the hot reality of cigarette smoke, mistaking the symbol for the thing symbolized. Language acts as a projection device, carrying the personal values of the language-user out into the territory (objects, persons, relationships, etc.) and giving the impression of modifying the territory. This impression is illusory.

The map is not *a map, but a mapping of the mapper mapping both himself and the territory.*
—J. S. BOIS, *BREEDS OF MEN*

Korzybski believed that the scientific method of careful, accurate observation, logical structuring of concepts, and an experimental view of experience could help to bring increased awareness to the nature of human thought, perception, and the use of symbol systems, such as language.

Further Resources

See resources for No. 10, Semantic awareness. For sixty-four years, the Institute for General Semantics has been hosting the presentation of the Alfred Korzybski Memorial Lecture. A complete list of the presentations is available at its website (generalsemantics.org). The Institute's journal is *ETC: A Review of General Semantics.*

• •

115 Final integration
Discovering your identity.

The term *final integration* is associated here with the theories of A. Reza Arasteh. Primarily a teacher and writer, Arasteh combines the theories of Western psychology with Eastern philosophical and spiritual teachings. He pays special attention to Sufi material familiar in his native Iran.

Arasteh points out that many industrial cultures make the dangerous and mistaken assumption that the individual has solved all problems of personal identity during adolescence. The identity crisis of adolescence is only a prelude to further identity crises where the questions of "Who am I?" and "Who are you?" must be answered. Arasteh feels that a solution to these adult identity problems can be achieved by a "final integration" in the adult personality.

A final integration necessitates a number of experiences, such as: new degrees of awareness, both internal and environmental; an anxious search for the truth, both personal and social; an existential moratorium, a period of time for maturation where one leaves oneself open and flexible to new views and experiences; intentional alienation from one's social role, or dropping out; an experience of liberation or transcendence where one's life gains meaning; and the experience of strong meaningful figures in one's life after returning to one's social group.

Further Resources

Arasteh's work is well presented in two books. *Rumi the Persian: Rebirth in Creativity and Love* examines the integrative process in thirteenth-century Persia through the study of a great Sufi poet and mystic. *Final Integration in the Adult Personality* is a clear-cut theoretical presentation of Arasteh's insights into the integrative process and its social applications through psychotherapy. In 2009, *The Journal of Transpersonal Psychology* published an updated appreciation of Arasteh's work by Joshua J. Knabb and Robert K. Welsh: "Reconsidering A. Reza Arasteh: Sufism and Psychotherapy."

• •

116 Thanatological awareness

Contemplating death brings about altered states.

Everyone who ever existed, everyone who exists now, has died or will die. This fact is very difficult to stay with, to make truly real. There are as many ways to rationalize death as there are to rob its eventuality of "realness."

When he was involved with psychedelics, Richard Alpert (Baba Ram Dass) suggested that a thanatology center be set up so that people could take psychedelics and learn about death—an idea that has gained greater traction recently with research into psychedelics and therapy for terminal illnesses. Though this is an interesting development, it is not altogether necessary to go to a center to learn about death. Most of us have known someone who is now dead, and most have lost someone close: parent, sibling, spouse, friend, or child.

The experience of the death of another can reveal new horizons to the living. Often, we think of the death of a relative or someone close solely as a negative experience. Death can be experienced in a very positive way. (This is not to discount the necessity for sadness and mourning over the dead; grief is a healthy emotion, in context.) The death of someone close can

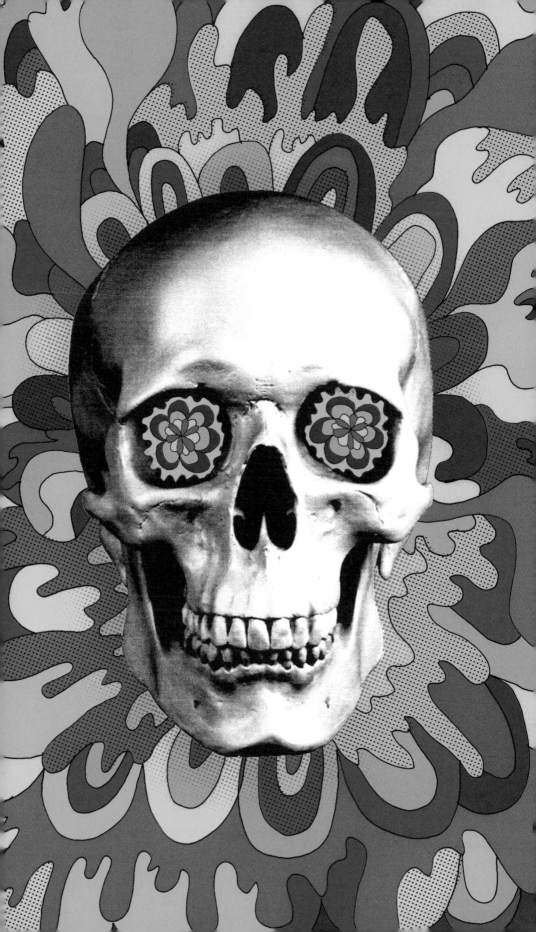

bring about a new view of life, a re-experiencing of life's very preciousness. Life can often be seen more clearly, and with new eyes, in the face of death.

Another positive aspect can come from the shock of impending death. Often people who are told that death is imminent totally change their attitudes toward life and their way of living.

And now she would have peace. And where there was peace and love, there too would be joy and the river of the colored lights was carrying her toward the white light of pure being, which is the source of all things and the reconciliation of all opposites in unity. . . . When the breathing ceased . . . it was without any struggle.
—ALDOUS HUXLEY, DESCRIBING THE DEATH OF HIS FIRST WIFE

Both the Egyptians and the Tibetans made elaborate preparations for death. The Egyptians made sure that the individual about to die would be well versed in how to behave in the next world and would have all of the tools needed there. The Tibetans treated dying as an art; a great deal of their wisdom has been preserved in the *Tibetan Book of the Dead.*

. . . the Art of Dying is quite as important as the Art of Living (or of Coming into Birth), of which it is the complement and summation.
—W. Y. EVANS-WENTZ, *THE TIBETAN BOOK OF THE DEAD*

With the recent rise of the Death Positivity movement, there has been an increasing number of death salons, gatherings to discuss death, even a death salon film festival. In addition, there have been more than 3,600 Death Cafes in more than thirty-seven countries.

On their mission, the lead organization, Death Salon, states:

> Death is sanitized and hidden in contemporary culture to the point of becoming a taboo subject. We aim to subvert this death denial by opening up conversations with the public about death and its anthropological, historical, and artistic contributions to culture. . . . Death Salon encourages conversations on mortality and mourning and their resonating effects on our culture and history . . . to increase discussion on this often-ignored subject, focusing more on ideas and the broader cultural impacts of death than one's personal interactions with mortality.

Further Resources

The Huxley quotation comes from the magnificent volume of his letters edited by Grover Smith. Consult the *Egyptian Book of the Dead* and W. Y. Evans-Wentz's rendering of *The Tibetan Book of the Dead.* Ram Dass, before he had an incapacitating stroke, served on the faculty of the Metta Institute, which is devoted to end-of-life issues. You can also learn more about Death Salon on their website (deathsalon.org) or their Twitter, Instagram, or Facebook accounts.

117 Gestalt therapy

Staying with the present: the here and now.

G estalt therapy was developed by Fritz Perls with his wife, Laura. Some believe it to be one of the most noteworthy clinical applications of psychology/philosophy since Freud.

The development of Gestalt therapy can be traced through seven major influences, all of which Perls brought to bear as he constantly changed, revised, and strengthened his clinical approach. These influences are:

1 Phenomenology and existentialism: Gestalt therapy is deeply rooted in phenomenological investigation. What Perls did was to turn from the existential question back to the phenomenological tool of the awareness continuum.

2 Gestalt psychology: Perls's work with the brain-injured, and with the great Gestalt psychologist Kurt Goldstein, did much to impress him with the pragmatic nature of Gestalt formulations of the interplay between figure and ground and with the theory of the self-actualizing organism.

3 Psychoanalysis: Perls spent most of his life fighting the shadow of Freud's powerful theories. Perls's analysis by Karen Horney, and later by Wilhelm Reich, plus interest in the work of Otto Rank, helped to guide and shape his own approach to psychotherapy.

4 Reich: In the work on the body Reich used in his character analysis, Perls found the unification that he had previously intuited was missing in psychoanalytic method.

5 Holism: While in South Africa, Perls had contact with the holistic theory of evolution of Jan Smuts. This helped to expand his view of the individual/organism-in-the-world.

6 General Semantics: Korzybski's work called attention to the all-important verbal level of the patient's world. Semantics aided the general phenomenological approach that Perls had already adopted.

7 Taoism/Zen Buddhism: These pragmatic mystical religions from the East enabled Perls to understand and complete the picture of the healthy Western human. From this picture emerged the human in relation to her/his true nature: freely being in the world in the here and now of the present moment.

The early development of Gestalt therapy started with the individual and his striving to complete his current unfinished situation in order to maintain a balance known as *homeostasis*. Perls paid special attention to the connection between hunger and aggression, discussing and theoretically examining the child's initial contact with food, the subsequent destructuring of the food, and the final digestion of nourishment achieved through this process that he considered a form of healthy aggression.

Also present in Perls's early work was the insistence on staying with the present, the here and now. Perls worked with projection (the patient's attempt to project onto others his own feelings), introjection (the patient's attempt to make something outside of him his own, often by "swallowing whole"), and retroflection (what the outside world bends back to the patient after he has directed it outward). From these insights and examinations came the realization that neurosis is a system of avoidance used by the patient to try to maintain some balance, often between his personal feelings and what he perceives as the world's (society's) dicta. Perls used as treatment a therapy based on concentration and awareness of the ongoing situation.

Perls used the Top Dog/Under Dog technique to bring about integration. Since Gestalt therapy did not use interpretative means, Perls felt that the I–Thou encounter (made famous by the work of theologian Martin Buber) could better make contact with the integrative forces. The Top Dog is the part of the self who is always saying "should" and who is always correct: "You should have called your mother. You know she'll be angry with you now. You've been a bad boy."

The Under Dog is the alternate self who confronts Top Dog: Under Dog is apologetic, manipulative, and usually the winner in any contest of the self: "I know I should have called; I'm sorry. I didn't mean to forget. I'll call tomorrow."

Perls also described three *shits:*

Chicken shit: The cliché talk of "hello, how are you, I'm fine, oh how nice." Most of this talk avoids real, meaningful contact.

Bull shit: Lies, exaggerations, stories, etc. "I'm the greatest (lover, talker, etc.) that ever lived." "I told him off."

Elephant shit: Theories, grand schemes, and explanations: ". . . the transcendental apperception which, through the essential mediation of the pure imagination, must be joined to pure intuition. . . ."

Perls defined maturity (in true "elephant-shit" fashion) as the transition from environmental support to self-support. When the patient can produce her own support for her own ventures and world actions, she is then operating as a mature and self-actualized organism.

Since Perls died, various practitioners have advanced, embellished, and complemented the Perlsian model of Gestalt therapy. Some more recent developments include: the integration of diagnosis into Gestalt therapy in the work of Elinor Greenberg; work to examine evidence-based work in Gestalt; the extension of Gestalt into relational and attachment paradigms, by Stella Resnick and (no relation) Rita and Robert Resnick.

Stella Resnick has also endeavored to unite insights from the neurosciences into her practice of Gestalt and her trainings. She cites four primary points:

1   Neurological rewiring for relearning.

2   The importance of play in setting up the capacity of the brain to rewire and to encourage neuroplasticity.

3   The importance of nonverbal communication to access different brain states and to undo hardwired brain states and brain chemistry.

4   The use of playful and nonverbal activities to affect neuroplasticity and neurochemistry.

Further Resources

The theoretical, practical, and experimental work of Gestalt therapy is available in Perls's books: *Ego, Hunger and Aggression* (the beginnings); *Gestalt Therapy* with Ralph Hefferline and Paul Goodman (the middle period); *Gestalt Therapy Verbatim* (the later work); and *In and Out the Garbage Pail* (an autobiography and history of the therapy). Elinor Greenberg's work on Gestalt diagnosis is described in "Borderline, Narcissistic, and Schizoid Adaptations: The Pursuit of Love, Admiration, and Safety" (2016) in P. Brownell & B. J. Mistler (Eds.) *Global Perspectives on Research, Theory, and Practice: A Decade of Gestalt!*. Stella Resnick's *The Heart of Desire: Keys to the Pleasures of Love* includes her integrations with Gestalt therapy. The very best theoretical (elephant shit) description and insight into Gestalt therapy comes from the second half of Perls, Hefferline, and Goodman. It was written by Paul Goodman based on the unpublished manuscripts of Perls.

. . . .

118 Maslovian psychology

To transcend, you must first satisfy basic needs.

M aslovian psychology encompasses the work of Abraham Maslow, who was basically a theoretical psychologist in that he did not develop a specific course of treatment for neurosis or psychosis. In fact, his most important contribution to the psychological sciences was his recognition that psychology was lacking a key perspective; one that had made most previous psychological contributions one-sided.

Maslow noted that all psychology was based on psychopathology, or the behavior and processes of sick people. Maslow decided that a new psychology was necessary, a psychology based on healthy people. He called these people *self-actualizers* (a term first used by the Gestalt psychologist Kurt Goldstein, with whom Maslow studied and worked). In order for someone to reach the highly developed states of consciousness that are self-actualization and, beyond that, self-transcendence, Maslow believed they had to satisfy different tiers of needs, starting with basics like food, love, and safety, then growth needs (e.g., knowledge, aesthetics), then self-actualization (fulfilling your potential), then self-transcendence (helping others, connecting with something beyond oneself). This became known as Maslow's Hierarchy of Needs.

A major aspect of the lives of these healthy people was their propensity to have what Maslow called peak experiences. Peak experiences are experiences of wonder, awe, ecstasy, altered consciousness, universal oneness, revelation, or transcendental states of being (see No. 90). With his studies of self-actualizers and their peak experiences, Maslow was able to help direct the attention of the psychological world toward developing methods of becoming healthy. This led to the development of Third Force or Humanistic Psychology (as opposed to the behavioristic or psychoanalytic models).

At the time of his death in 1970, Maslow was helping bring about the creation of a new psychology: " . . . A still higher Fourth Psychology, transpersonal, transhuman, centered in the cosmos rather than in human needs and interests. . . ." Though various aspects of transpersonal psychology have thrived in the years since Maslow's death (see No. 119), the "still higher Fourth Psychology" he envisioned is still awaiting a more substantial instantiation.

Further Resources

The work in his field by Abraham Maslow begins with *Motivation and Personality;* finds full development in *Toward a Psychology of Being;* and is further developed in *Religions, Values, and Peak-Experiences,* as well as numerous articles published in *The Journal of Humanistic Psychology* and *The Journal of Transpersonal Psychology.* Colin Wilson gives a detailed account of Maslow and Maslovian psychology in *New Pathways in Psychology: Maslow & the Post-Freudian Revolution.*

· ·

119 Transpersonal psychology

The spiritual psychology.

In the fevered ferment of the 1960s, when it seemed that everything new was replacing everything that was old, humanistic psychology forged new areas for development in individual and group therapies. During this same period, many of the same people seeking guidance from psychotherapeutic approaches were also reaching out on spiritual journeys of discovery, exploring new approaches to traditional Western religions, as well as Eastern religions, many previously thought of as too esoteric for Western sensibilities. As a result, transpersonal psychology came into practice, seeking to combine spiritual modalities within the framework of psychology.

Transpersonal psychology integrates the spiritual and transcendent aspects of the human experience with the framework of modern psychology. Many call transpersonal psychology the "spiritual" psychology. The British Psychological Society acknowledges this emphasis: "Transpersonal Psychology might loosely be called the psychology of spirituality and of those areas of the human mind which search for higher meanings in life, and which move beyond the limited boundaries of the ego to access an enhanced capacity for wisdom, creativity, unconditional love and compassion. It honors the existence of transpersonal experiences, and is concerned with their meaning for the individual and with their effect upon behavior."

Transpersonal psychology arose out of a feeling that humanistic psychology could be expanded and augmented. In 1967, there was a meeting with humanistic psychology pioneers Abraham Maslow, Anthony Sutich, and others to create what they hoped would be a new, more spiritual approach to psychology. What followed was the founding of the Association of Transpersonal Psychology and the start of the *Journal of Transpersonal Psychology*.

Stanislav Grof also addresses the important aspects of psychology that the transpersonal approach makes possible:

> Transpersonal psychology has made a significant headway toward correcting the ethnocentric and cognicentric bias of mainstream psychiatry and psychology, particularly by its recognition of the genuine nature of transpersonal experiences and their value. In the light of modern consciousness research, the current conceited dismissal and pathologization of spirituality characteristic of monistic materialism appears untenable. The spiritual dimensions of reality can be directly experienced in a way that is as convincing as our daily experience of the material world, if not more so. Careful study of transpersonal experiences shows that they cannot be explained as products of pathological processes in the brain, but are ontologically real.

Further Resources

Grof's history of transpersonal psychology can be found on his website (stanislavgrof.com). The Association for Transpersonal Psychology also provides abundant resources on its website (atpweb.org). A contemporary video by Charles Tart, author of *Transpersonal Psychologies*, can be found on *The Book of Highs* YouTube playlist.

• •

120 Sensory training

The re-education of your senses.

Sensory training refers to the work of Charlotte Selver and Charles V. W. Brooks. Their work, in turn, is based upon the formulations of Elsa Gindler and Heinrich Jacoby. Sensory training involves the re-education of the senses. Today, with so much going on in the environment, our senses are often overloaded. In order to cope, we shut down our sensory equipment so that we receive a minimum amount of sensory input. This is an attempt to cut out the noises, the blaring colors of advertisements, and the conditions brought on by urban overcrowding.

The idea of sensory training is to bring people back to their senses so that they may appreciate all of the wonderful sensations available to them.

Selver and Brooks's approach starts by having people lie on the floor. The attempt is then made to help individuals return to original perceptions.

Distinction between inside and outside (the floor touches me; I touch the floor); right and wrong; watching and looking; thinking and experiencing are relearned. This is known as "inner awakening."

After this has progressed, the work on balancing begins. Again natural positions and activities—lying, sitting, standing, and walking—are used for relearning experiences. These involve sensing the differences between habit and coordination; noting the constants of change and flux; and awakening to the entire environment.

We find ourselves being more one with the world where we formerly had to cross barriers. Thoughts and ideas "come" in lucidity instead of being produced. We don't have to try to express ourselves (as the word so vividly depicts), but utterances become just part of the natural functioning. Experiences can be allowed to be more fully received and to mature in us.
—SELVER AND BROOKS

Further Resources

Some references for this work are given in the resource material for No. 4. A good description of a Selver workshop is included in *Turning On* by Rasa Gustaitis. Selver taught this workshop up until her death in 2003. Sensory training has been embraced by those working in diverse disciplines, ranging from food and beer to working with autistic and elderly populations.

• •

121 Bio-energetic analysis

Breathing and body exercises for healing and greater peace.

Bio-energetics is a continuation of the character-analysis and body-armor work of Wilhelm Reich. This extension has been pursued mostly by Alexander Lowen and John Pierrakos.

Bio-energetics deals with the person as body. It emphasizes the fact that we *are* our bodies; we do not *have* bodies. It deals with the body on a number of levels, including shape, flexibility, rigidity, blocks, and total body form and expression. As with Reich's character armor, Lowen believed that our psychological defenses could manifest as mental health and muscular problems. To fix this tension, bio-energetics uses a system of breathing and body exercises and psychological therapy.

We have no real existence apart from our bodies. What goes on in our minds is, basically, a reflection of what goes on in our bodies.
—ALEXANDER LOWEN

Bio-energetics seeks to reintegrate man with five very recognizable realizations. The first is to reestablish the individual's identification with his body. The second is the recognition of the pleasure principle as the basis for consciousness experience. The third is to accept, to *be*, one's feelings. The fourth is to know that all awareness is subjective awareness. This allows for objectivity when the subjectivity of consciousness is acknowledged. The fifth is humility. Humility is the recognition of ultimate powerlessness in the cosmos. It knows that neither humbleness nor arrogance is the answer, but that realization of the uniqueness of individuality leads to true grounding in reality.

Lowen devised a number of postures and exercises that he felt would help the individual on a path of natural healing. These include the two body bows, stretching backward and bending over forward; arching the back over a stool; and the hyperextensionized body circle. These passive positions help the individual experience the body and the areas of tension. They add dynamics and help liberate new energy.

Lowen followed these with a number of active movements. The first active position is striking: You can strike a bed with a tennis racket or with your fists. In the second active movement, the individual kicks the bed while lying on his or her back. The bed may be kicked with legs bent or extended. Flailing of the arms may accompany the kicking.

These exercises and postures enable the individual to breathe and then translate that breathing into action.

Further Resources

The principal exposition of bio-energetic theory is in two of Lowen's books, *The Betrayal of the Body* (which includes detailed descriptions of the bio-energetic exercises) and *Pleasure*. Lowen died in 2008, just shy of his ninety-eighth birthday. His work is being continued by the International Institute for Bioenergetic Analysis (bioenergetic-therapy.com).

122 Grounding and energy

How does your body receive, transform, and distribute energy?

The term "grounding" is used here to describe the work of Stanley Keleman. Keleman reunifies people with their animal origins so that they will then be able to *be* their bodies, to experience the flow of energy through the body, and to experience being grounded. Keleman says:

> To me, grounding means being anchored in our physical-psychic growth processes: expanding, contracting (contact, withdrawal), charging, discharging. . . . The opposite of grounding is flight, or interference with our human essence; its products (our common ailments) are fear, rage, frustration and dissatisfaction. Separation from the biological ground results in anguish and despair instead of the great potential for vitality, love, contact and growth with which we have been endowed.

Seeing the human animal as an energy system, Keleman recognizes three ways in which the body accepts, transforms, and redistributes different forms of energy, through discharge. First, the energy that moves from the head toward the earth. Interference releases unsureness, doubt and anxiety. Second, the build-up and discharge of tension on the part of the body: expansion and contraction. Interference here produces frustration, anger, and despair. Finally, there is sexual energy centered in the lower section of the body. Interference here produces immobility and panic.

Grounding enables the patient to become aware of tensions, blocks, splits, and interferences and thus deepens world contact and available energy, increasing feeling, while helping them learn to live with the heightened awareness.

In his therapy and workshops with groups, Keleman uses repetition tapes (see No. 241) to establish a time-kaleidoscoped system of deprogramming. In one exercise, Keleman lets the group hear everyday demands and commands ("Don't do that") many thousands of times in several hours. As we grow up, we hear these commands that many times only in a number of years. He plays these tapes while the group members experience increased energetic charges through the use of the exercises devised by Alexander Lowen (No. 121). What then occurs is that the mind and body respond by lifting out old memories and new possibilities and the individuals take possession of their bodies. This technique changes the psychological and physiological status of the individual.

While this is occurring, Keleman often uses a tape with a positive universal program ("You and I are one"). To another track on the tape, he often adds music that he feels supplies the equivalent of background neural noise (e.g., Terry Riley's *In C*) and then has the group lie or sit in a circle, holding hands or putting their feet together. This leads to a variety of cosmic experiences, including visions, hallucinations, out-of-body experiences, and mythic journeys.

Keleman finds that the intensity of these techniques increases with the size of the group.

Further Resources

This information was drawn from a personal communication with Keleman and two pamphlets. One, titled "The Body Groups and Consciousness" is available through the growth center, Kairos. The other, "Bio-Energetic Concepts of Grounding" was published by Lodestar Press (it's available at openlibrary.org). *Sexuality, Self and Survival* has been produced from edited recordings of several Keleman workshops. Keleman, who still practices in Berkeley, California, now calls his approach to body work and education Formative Psychology. His Center for Energetic Studies has an extensive collection of his books and recordings. Keleman was heavily influenced by his mentor, Nina Bull, another pioneer in the field of body psychotherapy. See her books, *Attitude Theory of Emotions* and *The Body and Its Mind.*

• •

123 Psychomotor therapy

Processing emotions and memories through movement and reenactment.

Psychomotor therapy refers to the techniques of psychotherapy and movement developed by Albert Pesso (1929–2016), a professional dancer, a teacher of dance, and a choreographer. It is a largely nonverbal technique teaching patients to be aware of their emotions and the expression of emotional impulses.

Pesso's technique revolves around a group that can come together regularly under the guidance of a therapist trained in psychomotor therapy. The work of the group proceeds through three stages. In the first stage, the group is presented with sensitization of motor impulses. This is achieved through learning how to stand and through such exercises as proper stance (a "species stance," a stance of complete relaxation in which the head droops, arms hang loose, and the body is kept upright by reflex rather than conscious tension), raising the arms in the stance, a torso twist, and basic walks.

The second stage deals with the enactment of specific emotional situations, often a reliving of a traumatic experience. The group acts as "accommodators" by giving the expected and appropriate response to the individual's enactment.

In the third stage, the emotions and their functional expressions are polarized into positive and negative configurations. This too is achieved through group responses. The bad figures (played by group members) represent the bad aspects of real life and often provide the opportunity for cathartic release. The positive figures (also played by group members) represent the desired goals, the ideals of real life, and facilitate the replacement of frustrating and often harmful experiences.

Further Resources

Pesso's *Movement in Psychotherapy* outlines his methods and describes group procedures. The Pesso-Boyden System Psychomotor Institute's website (pbsp.com) also provides helpful information on practitioners and research. Bessel van der Kolk's *The Body Keeps the Score* describes the application of psychomotor techniques to soldiers, police, firefighters, and others exposed to excessive stress and trauma. *The New York Times Magazine* published an article discussing van der Kolk's work, "A Revolutionary Approach to Treating PTSD," on May 25, 2014.

124 Psychosynthesis

Finding the core of the self via hypnosis and visualization.

Psychosynthesis is a system developed over more than half a century by Robert Assagioli. It is concerned with the separate and separative elements of the psyche. It postulates that there is an unchanging "I-consciousness." Unlike physical-emotional-biological-mental states that change constantly and consistently, this "I-consciousness" is a persistent central core of the self.

In order to reach this unifying center of the self, Assagioli developed methods for self-identification awareness, strengthening the will, and visualization. All of these revolve around imaginative evocations. There are certain key phrases, similar to hypnotic inductions, that are repeated and experienced. Symbols, colors, programmed daydreams, and a variety of other techniques are used in this treatment.

Assagioli and his associates developed and described more than forty separate techniques of psychosynthesis. Following is a description of the technique of visualization:

> First, imagine the setting, which is a classroom with a blackboard, gray or dull black. Then imagine that in the middle of the blackboard appears a figure; let us say the number five, as if written with white chalk, fairly large and well defined. Then keep it vividly before your inner eye, so to speak; that is, keep the image of the five vivid and steady in the field of your conscious attention. Then on the right of the five visualize the figure two.
>
> So, now you have two figures, a five and a two, making fifty-two. Dwell for a while on the visualization of this number, then after a little while, imagine the appearance of a four at the right side of the two.
>
> Now you have three figures, written in white chalk, five, two, four—making the number five hundred and twenty-four. Dwell for a while on this number.
>
> Continue adding other figures until you are unable to hold together the visualization of the number resulting from those figures.

Further Resources

A book named for the method, *Psychosynthesis,* outlines Robert Assagioli's principles and techniques. It also includes a bibliography of his publications. The archives of the Psychosynthesis Research Foundation can be found at psychosynthesisresources.com. Other monographs and articles about psychosynthesis can be found at synthesiscenter.org. The most important recent book on psychosynthesis is *Psychosynthesis: A Psychology of the Spirit* by John Firman and Ann Gila.

125 Client-centered therapy

Reflecting someone's feelings back at them can lead to greater awareness.

Client-centered therapy was one of the first American attempts at an existential, humanistic psychology. The approach was developed by Carl Rogers, who constantly and consistently centered the therapy around the experience of the patient by offering him phenomenological feedback of what he had just described to the therapist.

An example through dialogue will illustrate:

Patient: My wife made me so mad this morning.

Therapist: You're angry with your wife for something she did.

Patient: Yes, she forgot to take my shirts to the laundry. She did it deliberately because I ignored her.

Therapist: I see. Your wife forgot your shirts on purpose, to punish you for not paying proper attention to her.

In this way the patient is exposed to how he is reporting his experience, and thereby can gain insight into his own behavior. Rogers believed that people were inherently good and that if you provided them with "unconditional positive regard" and reflected back to them what they were doing, they'd have insight into how to be a better person, because we all ultimately just want to be good in the world.

Further Resources

Rogers's books, *Counseling and Psychotherapy* and *Client-Centered Therapy,* spell out the basics of his approach. His later work is described in his *On Becoming a Person, Freedom to Learn,* and *Person to Person* by Rogers and Barry Stevens. The film *Three Approaches to Psychotherapy* devotes time to three psychotherapeutic interviews with the same female patient. Rogers, Albert Ellis (Rational Psychotherapy), and Fritz Perls (Gestalt therapy) show their techniques. The film is available on YouTube (search for "Three approaches to psychotherapy" or "the Gloria films," so named for the patient).

126 Behavior therapy

We cannot study how someone *thinks*, but we can study how someone *behaves*.

B ehavior therapy maintains that there is no way to truly know what occurs in one's mind, so we must examine only the observable behavior of the patient. By treating the symptom—that is, by helping the patient unlearn old types of behavior responsible for the symptom, and by helping them develop new ways of adapting—the neurosis is cured.

Behavior therapy holds that a series of hierarchies of anxiety is built up by the patient. To deal with these psychological structures, two basic techniques are used by therapists.

In the first technique, the patient learns to relax by tensing each part of the musculature separately. After holding the tense position for some time, he completely relaxes the area just tensed. The entire body is worked on in this way with the therapist determining when relaxation is achieved. Following this instruction, the patient is usually capable of achieving a form of total body relaxation.

In the second technique, the patient is encouraged to fantasize a scene that relates in some way to his self-described symptoms. When the therapist senses that the patient is experiencing anxiety, he encourages him to develop the fantasy, and then instructs him to relax totally. After relaxation is achieved, the patient returns to the fantasy. Eventually anxiety is reduced.

Behavior therapy also uses other methods, including aversion therapy (punishment during exposure to symbols of the neurotic behavior), operant conditioning of both the positive and the negative type, and rewarding of assertive behavior.

Operant conditioning, formulated by B. F. Skinner, has two basic premises: one, to reward correct behavior by positive reinforcement, and two, the instruction of desirable behavior patterns in small, slow steps. Assertive behavior is usually rewarded by verbal approval and reinforcement from the therapist. The types of negative conditioning used range from verbal threats and castigation to the use of certain forms of electric shock, and have proved to be harmful.

Further Resources

T he primary text in this field is *Behavior Therapy Techniques* by J. Wolpe and A. A. Lazarus. A good introduction to the technique is available in Beech's *Changing Man's Behavior*. It has a bibliography with almost 150 entries for further reading.

....

127 Cognitive behavioral therapy

How realistic are your thoughts and perceptions?

D eveloped by Aaron Beck along with his daughter, Judith, cognitive behavioral therapy (CBT) is just like the words indicate: a therapy, based on cognition and thinking, and contrasting that thinking with behavior and actions. From the Beck Institute's website: "CBT is a psychotherapy that is based on the cognitive model: The way that individuals perceive a situation is more closely connected to their reaction than the situation itself. An important part of CBT is helping clients change their unhelpful thinking and behavior that lead to enduring improvement in their mood and functioning."

CBT uses a variety of cognitive and behavioral techniques, but it isn't defined by its use of these strategies. Practitioners borrow from many psychotherapeutic modalities, including dialectical behavior therapy, acceptance and commitment therapy, Gestalt therapy, compassion-focused therapy, mindfulness, solution-focused therapy, motivational interviewing, positive psychology, interpersonal psychotherapy, and when it comes to personality disorders, psychodynamic psychotherapy.

The Foundation for Cognitive Therapy and Research describes four key terms that are essential in the practice of CBT: Cognitive formulation—the beliefs and behavioral strategies that characterize a specific disorder. Conceptualization—understanding of individual clients and their specific beliefs or patterns of behavior. Cognitive model—the idea that the way that individuals perceive a situation is more closely connected to their reaction than the situation itself. Automatic thoughts—ideas that seem to pop up in your mind.

Judith Beck describes the therapy in this way: "CBT helps people identify their distressing thoughts and evaluate how realistic the thoughts are. Then they learn to change their distorted thinking. When they think more realistically, they feel better. The emphasis is also consistently on solving problems and initiating behavioral change."

As a result of feeling better and thinking better, people find that the behavioral changes from cognitive behavioral therapy can bring about lasting transformations of consciousness. Experiences are often new and different once new ways of thinking and behaving are integrated into daily life.

Further Resources

T he Beck Institute has a variety of useful resources, including the Q & A from Judith Beck quoted above (beckinstitute.org). PsychCentral (psychcentral.com) has a good introductory essay on CBT by Ben Martin. For a good introduction to CBT as a patient, see *Feeling Good: The New Mood Therapy* by David D. Burns.

• •

128 Eye movement desensitization and reprocessing

How rapid eye movements can help us process trauma.

S tress, trauma, and other seeming constants of twenty-first-century life can be overwhelming. A series of treatments and therapeutic approaches have emerged in order to deal with these ills of the mind and body. These therapies include treatments for post-traumatic stress disorders (PTSD), automobile and other transportation-related accidents, death and the loss of family and loved ones, and so many more stress-filled experiences.

An important therapeutic approach to these ills is eye movement desensitization and reprocessing. As the patient relives the traumatic experience, the therapist moves her hand back in forth in front of him, causing him to follow the hand with rapid eye movements. In conjunction with the movement the therapist guides the patient in reframing the trauma (e.g., replacing negative thoughts with positive ones), leading to emotional transformations and the encouragement of new coping skills to deal with the painful event.

Why do the eye movements work? There are many theories—perhaps it's the soothing effect of repetitive motion. Or is it the syncing of the brain's hemispheres? Or maybe it's how the movement mimics the rapid eye movement (REM) of sleep. More research is needed.

Further Resources

T he EMDR Institute (emdr.com) has helpful information and resources about that therapeutic approach.

. . . .

129 Encounter
Baring yourself in the group.

The word "encounter" was first used in relation to group therapy by J. L. Moreno (see No. 110) in 1912. Carl Rogers called these psychotherapy groups "the basic encounter group," and the name stuck. But it was only in the 1960s and 1970s that encounter groups gained wide popularity.

Briefly, encounter signifies the attempt by a group, with a leader or without, to meet and experience each other as real individuals, without masks, roles, or protective games. This means that many will have to drop their defenses. They will have to stand before the group, with all of their faults and deficiencies on display. For some individuals this means an opportunity to find new strengths, to use potential abilities untapped in the workaday world, to find and/or to give support, and to experience crisis and growth in a safe environment.

Encounter groups present a safe environment in which to experiment with taking chances, to try out involvement, feeling, and the expression of emotions. With this experience can come the development of facilities for trusting.

By trying out these experiences in the safety of the encounter group, by taking chances where support is forthcoming, the individual will, it is hoped, gain self-assurance and be able to extend their strengths into the world at large.

Although the encounter approach has faded from use, self-help groups who meet regularly to discuss grief, addiction, loneliness, and other mental health issues still employ its exercises and strategies. As Irvin Yalom says in his updated edition of *The Theory and Practice of Group Psychotherapy*, "though the encounter group movement is dead and buried, the sophisticated technology of the encounter group persists and is widely employed by groups that are very much alive. . . . So, although the movement is over and an encounter group *qua* encounter group is hard to find, more people than ever before are having an encounter group experience."

Further Resources

Encounter technique is described in several essays in H. Otto and J. Mann's *Ways of Growth*, in Schutz's *Joy*, and in Hendrik Ruitenbeek's *The New Group Therapies*. A basic text showing the origins of this method is Bradford, Gibb, and Benne's *T-Group Theory and Laboratory Method*. The Yalom quotation comes from *The Theory and Practice of Group Psychotherapy*, which also discusses encounter groups.

130 Marathon

Long-form group therapy.

M arathon was devised by George R. Bach as an extension of the encounter process. It is a very simple procedure. A group meets in an encounter situation, but instead of breaking up after three, six, or eight hours, they continue to stay together, exploring in a variety of different ways, for as long as fourteen hours. Sometimes groups will stay together for a full twenty-four hours. The usual schedule is to meet for fourteen hours, part to sleep, meet again for another fourteen hours, and disband.

Staying with a group for a long period of time, where human interaction is as direct, spontaneous, open, and honest as is possible, can be taxing on defense systems after only an hour or two. After ten hours, most defenses have been stripped away.

Further Resources

R uitenbeek's chapter "The Encounter Marathon" is one of the best in his book *The New Group Therapies*; the book also has many references to other articles. Another of his books, *Group Therapy Today,* reprints some important comments on marathon, including a paper by its founder, Bach. In 2002, the *Consulting Psychology Journal* published a look back at the practice titled "The Marathon Encounter Group—Vision and Reality: Exhuming the Body for a Last Look" by Richard G. Weigel.

131 Potentials

Tapping old and new sources of sensory, familial, and creative energy.

T he term *potentials* refers here to the work in psychotherapeutic processes developed by Herbert Otto to bring people into better contact with the potential abilities and emotions they possess but do not use. While potentials certainly had its heyday during the '60s and '70s, especially at institutes like Esalen, these exercises aren't used as often today. Here are a few of Otto's key interventions for tapping into one's potentials:

Sensory restimulation: With a system similar to the sensory training done by Selver, Brooks, and Gunther (No. 4 and No. 120), Otto advocated that sensory awakening experiments be done not for "kicks" but for "affirmation."

The inventory technique: The family gathers and takes an inventory of its specific strengths and weaknesses as a group. Members of the family support the person reporting and help to make him or her aware of things overlooked. Assignments can be given in order to follow up on material that is uncovered during the inventory, with an agreement to meet again for reassessment

Strength bombardment: One family member is selected and the others "bombard" him or her with verbal reports of the individual's strengths and assets in relation to the family.

The Minerva experience: Otto describes the Minerva experience as a positive, creative past experience associated with deep emotional feelings. These experiences alter and affect the way the individual grows and develops potentials. By uncovering and recalling these experiences, the individual can tap old *and* new sources of psychic energy. The Minerva experience may also free creative potential that is applicable to current life situations.

Further Resources

Two books edited by Otto, *Explorations in Human Potentialities* and *Ways of Growth* (with John Mann as coeditor), contain a number of his papers. The *Explorations* book gives references for further reading.

• •

132 Art therapy
Healing through creating.

A few hours alone or with friends with a box of paints, pens, crayons, or finger paints can be one of the simplest and most interesting techniques for altering consciousness.

In art therapy, the object is to provide the patient with a nonverbal techniques for freeing their feelings and affirming them through a medium of self-expression. In addition, it can often allow hidden talent to be exposed. In a group, if all the members are engaged in the production of a single work, it may be even easier for the individual to expose their inner feelings. Art therapy can be used to treat blocks and unresolved problems as well as problems of identity and creativity.

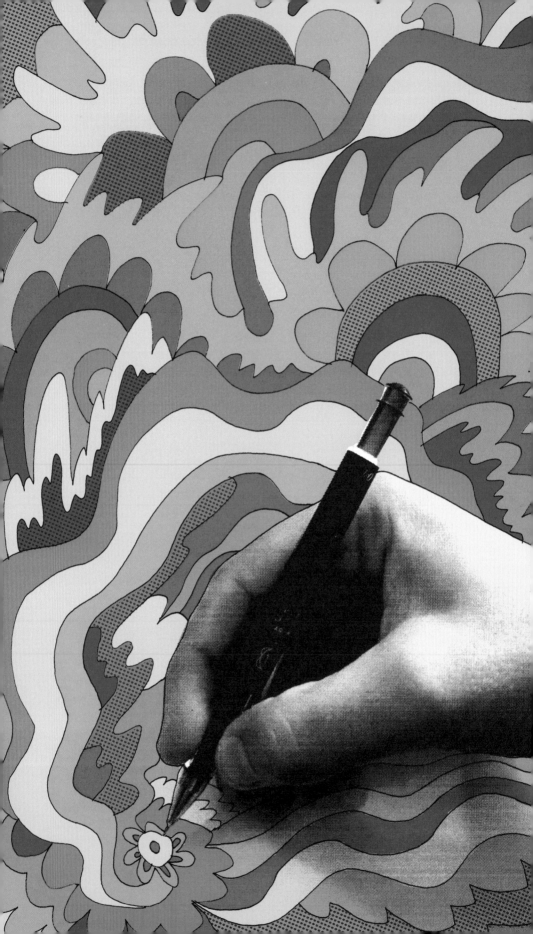

Janie Rhyne (1913–1995) pioneered the combination of Gestalt therapy and art therapy. She introduced some of her groups by having each member do something with a selected medium, such as clay, chalks, finger paint, and so on. What is stressed, once the artworks are in process, is that you are the work of art that you create; the work is an extension of your self.

Another exercise involves breaking a group down into subgroups of five (a nucleus, and North, South, East, and West). These five are told that they are the only people left on the planet and are then urged to design and create their own community, in models.

Experiments such as these make art therapy a vehicle for nonverbal self-discovery and consciousness enhancement.

Further Resources

Consult the American Art Therapy Association (arttherapy.org).

133 Family therapy

Reassessing family roles is "thinking the unthinkable."

Family therapy is practiced by any number of therapists. Probably the best known is Virginia Satir, who called her approach "conjoint family therapy." In conjoint family therapy she stressed the various aspects of communication—verbal, nonverbal, and sensory—as well as the problems of having close but free relationships. In her workshops she synthesized a variety of techniques including sensory awakening, encounter (No. 129), and role-playing to strengthen perception and awareness of family abilities.

She also established what she called "well-family" clinics throughout the United States to stress and aid in the fostering of positive family functioning. Often, the reevaluation of family roles, rules, and relationships is referred to as "thinking about the unthinkable," since the very core and structure of family ties can be threatened by exposure and examination. But most often, the family that can expose its inner cares, order, and workings to thorough evaluation benefits through the development of more flexibility and interchange between the different family members.

Satir stressed reconsidering our roles in the family unit and how it impacts the way we react and respond to stress and conflict later in life. It might seem "unthinkable" to cast aside your family role, but it is how you will find your authentic self.

Further Resources

Satir outlined her theories and practice in *Conjoint Family Therapy*. The Ackerman Institute (ackerman.org) has many resources connected to family therapy approaches.

• •

134 A Psychobiological Approach to Couple Therapy (PACT)

Neuroscience, attachment theory, and the biology of human arousal.

One of the most important developments in psychotherapeutic work with couples is the approach developed and pioneered by Stan Tatkin. He calls his work PACT—A Psychobiological Approach to Couple Therapy, and in it he integrates, among other approaches, aspects of discoveries from the neurosciences with attachment theory and the enhancement of arousal regulation.

According to Tatkin, PACT draws from three areas:

The first is neuroscience, the study of the human brain. Understanding how the brain works provides a physiological basis for understanding how people act and react within relationships. In a nutshell, some areas of your brain are wired to reduce threat and danger and seek security, while others are geared to establish mutuality and loving connection.

The second is attachment theory, which explains the biological need to bond with others. Experiences in early relationships create a blueprint that informs the sense of safety and security you bring to adult relationships. Insecurities that have been carried through life can wreak havoc for a couple if these issues are not resolved.

The third area is the biology of human arousal—meaning the moment-to-moment ability to manage one's energy, alertness, and readiness to engage. It isn't necessary to understand the scientific basis of PACT to realize its benefits.

Tatkin notes that the key features of his PACT approach include focusing on shifts in your body and voice (both as an individual and as a couple) while also working through troubling issues in the relationship. The sessions can be lengthy—lasting as long as three to six hours—but, according to Tatkin, PACT often requires fewer sessions than other forms of couple therapy.

Further Resources

For more information, see Tatkin's PACT website (stantatkin.com).

• •

135 Dance therapy
Self-awareness and self-discovery through dance.

Dance therapy was originally formulated by Marian Chace as a means for dealing with catatonic veterans who were hospitalized following World War II. Her initial discovery was that these patients could be temporarily lifted out of their catatonic state by starting to dance. If they could be enticed to dance, they were then encouraged to form a circle. As they danced and started to move their pelvic regions, their eyes would begin to come back into focus.

As a result of the dancing, many of the patients began wanting to get well and would, for the first time, become amenable to help from the psychiatric staff.

Later, Chace trained dancers to do dance therapy in mental hospitals, and before her death she was able to open up nearly every psychiatric hospital to dance, where before there had been none.

Dance therapy is very similar to movement in therapy. The aim is to help the individual find a means of self-expression and of integrating movement.

Generally, dance therapy takes two forms. Some groups operate around a series of set movements that are practiced until they can be executed to the satisfaction of both patient and therapist; they may be individual movements or a programmed sequence.

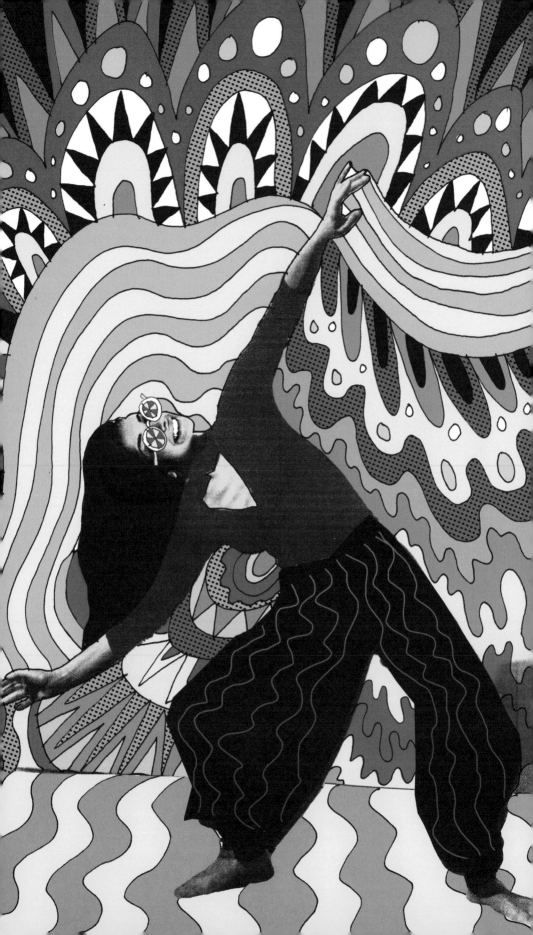

The second type of dance therapy group emphasizes free-form discovery. Different types of music are played and the patient is encouraged to try out spontaneous expression of body position and varied movements that fit the music, the environment, and the patient's feelings and ongoing experience. The aim is toward self-awareness through the discovery of personal spontaneity and style.

What can be particularly exciting in dance therapy is the discovery of some new form of self-expression. Often the leader will request that the dance form be used to express the emotions between group members.

What we do while dancing is often more honest and direct than what we do verbally in day-to-day contact.

Further Resources

See the *American Journal of Dance Therapy* as well as the website for the American Dance Therapy Association (adta.org).

136 Imago relationship therapy

What is your unconscious image of love?

Ask any psychotherapist, psychologist, or psychiatrist about what kinds of therapy present the most challenges and many will respond, "treating couples in their relationship with each other." Imago relationship therapy (IRT) provided a breakthrough approach to working with couples, emphasizing and focusing on the couple's relationship as a separate entity from each of the couple as individuals. It was co-developed by Harville Hendrix and his wife, Helen LaKelly Hunt, and documented in Hendrix's 1988 book, *Getting the Love You Want, A Guide for Couples*. That book was featured on Oprah Winfrey's TV show and catapulted Hendrix into the public spotlight as Winfrey's favored therapist (that is, until Oprah found Dr. Phil).

The term *imago* is Latin for "image" and refers to the "unconscious image of familiar love." Simply put, there is often a connection between the frustrations experienced in adult relationships and early childhood experiences. If you frequently felt criticized as a child, you will likely be sensitive to any criticism from your partner and feel criticized more often by him or her. If you felt abandoned, smothered, neglected, etc., these feelings will also often arise in your marriage or your committed relationships.

Most people face only a few of these core issues, but they often arise again and again within partnerships. This can overshadow all that is good in the relationship, leaving people to wonder if they have chosen the right mate. When you can understand your partner's feelings and empathize with their childhood wounds, you can begin to heal yourself and your relationship, and move toward a more conscious relationship.

IRT can help this process by teaching couples the Imago Dialogue process, where partners listen to what their mate says and then reflect back what they heard. This often reveals how couples do and do not listen and pay attention to each other, most especially if their partner's wounds touch areas where they themselves have been and are wounded. The dialogue process can then help couples to move from blame and reactivity to understanding and empathy. With this dialogue process the couple can transform conflicts into opportunities for healing and growth, and connect more deeply and lovingly with their partners for increased intimacy in the relationship.

By experiencing another's wounds, couples can come together, holding each other for the first time in this new way, with an altered and expanded awareness of their partner.

Further Resources

In addition to Hendrix's 1988 book, he and Hunt have published numerous works, including *Keeping the Love You Find: A Personal Guide*, *Making Marriage Simple*, and *Receiving Love*. Imago Relationships International also provides valuable resources (imagorelationships.org).

• •

137 Theater games
Improvising and experimenting.

Theater games are a result of the application of the principles of psychodrama (See No. 110) to therapeutic and political situations. Street theater, guerilla theater, The Committee on the West Coast (1963–1972) and La MaMa E.T.C. (1961–the present: lamama.org) on the East Coast are examples of the political aspects of theater games in action.

The therapeutic approach to theater games was pioneered by Viola Spolin (1906–1994). She describes a number of strategies in the form of theatrical "games" that groups can play together. Some examples:

One member of the group assumes a position on the floor. The other members of the group are told to link up to him, one by one, to form a machine, with moving, working parts.

Three members of a group are picked to tell a story. But none of them knows what the story is, how it begins, proceeds, or ends. The story is determined by the three improvising with one another.

The whole group is told to tell a story. Each member tells part of the story and the person next to him has to pick up where he stops, even if it is in midsentence, without a pause of more than three seconds.

Further Resources

Improvisations for the Theater by Viola Spolin is the main work in the field. In it she makes reference to other writers.

138 Primal therapy

A controversial approach to reliving childhood trauma through screaming.

Primal therapy was developed by Arthur Janov (1924–2017). Janov claims that the primal therapy technique is not only the cure for neurosis and psychosis but for a variety of other ailments. By recalling and reliving repressed childhood trauma, the patient would experience his primal pain usually via screaming or hysteria, and eventually reach a kind of catharsis.

> Painful things happen to nearly all of us early in life that get imprinted in all our systems which carry the memory forward, making our lives miserable. It is the cause of depression, phobias, panic, and anxiety attacks and a whole host of symptoms that add to the misery. We have found a way into those early emotional archives and have learned to have access to those memories, to dredge them up from the unconscious, allowing us to re-experience them in the present, integrate them and no longer be driven by the unconscious.

Primal therapy, or primaling, starts when the prospective patient is accepted by the primal therapist on the basis of an autobiographical account. No personal interview is conducted. Next comes a thorough medical examination to ensure that the patient is physically sound enough to withstand the rigors of primaling. Then the patient is isolated for twenty-four to forty-eight hours. Any contact with outsiders, media (including reading material), drugs (including tobacco and alcohol) is prohibited. This isolation lowers the patient's defenses. The patient then begins a three-week period where he is the only patient seen by the therapist. The course of therapy might well be called "pain encounter." In sessions lasting as long as twelve hours, the patient is told to relive their life, and goes back into their past to recount all of their painful experiences, often including a fantasy re-experiencing of childbirth itself. Janov claims that through the patient's contact with pain, the primal pains (the pains experienced in childhood) will eventually appear. With the primal pains come the primal screams for "mommy" and "daddy."

After three weeks of individual sessions, the patient moves on to group primal experience, three-hour sessions that take place twice a week and can go on for several months. Twenty to fifty or so patients make up the group. At the completion of the group experience the patient is "cured."

It should be noted that primal therapy lacks significant clinical research to support it and in some cases has made patients worse. Should you decide to try primal therapy, proceed with care.

Further Resources

Primal Therapy is the name of Janov's first book, detailing his therapeutic approach and procedures. The quote is from an article, "The Primal Doctor" by Jerry Hopkins, which appeared in *Rolling Stone* (February 18, 1971). Janov's latest published books are titled *The Anatomy of Mental Illness* and *The Primal Revolution*. The Janov Primal Center is located in Santa Monica, CA (primaltherapy.com).

• •

139 Rolfing

Free your body for new ways of moving.

Rolfing, or structural integration, takes its name from Ida Rolf (1896–1979), who developed this system of deep-muscle manipulation and realignment. In Rolfing, the practitioner focuses on the client's body and the physical manifestations of the body's relationship to gravity and the environment. A Rolfer analyzes the interplay of structure, movement, energy, and tension in the way the client lives in the environment and helps the client to free his body for new ways of moving.

Rolfing teaches that the client's body is a mirror of past experience and will display the damage resulting from emotional experience as well as physical trauma. Experiences from early childhood are often reflected in the posture and carriage of the adult.

Your body reacts to a variety of stimuli with tension, rigidity, and resistance. These reactions eventually bring about a habitual muscle position because the muscle sheaths, or fascia, lock and control muscle movement and tone. Once the fascia become rigidified, it is almost impossible to change muscle position at will. All the mothers in the world telling Johnny to stand up straight won't help. Johnny can temporarily pull his shoulders back, but he's already fixed into contracting his diaphragm as a habitual response to situations of anxiety and stress.

The Rolfer works with the client by reaching in and realigning the muscle fascia so that body structure may be reintegrated, with special attention paid to gravity and the client's contact with and grounding to the earth.

Rolfers claim that work on a client can be completed after as little as ten hours of structural integration work. The result is new freedom in posture, alignment, muscle tone, and usage. This can be accompanied by a reduction of tension.

A frequent complaint associated with Rolfing is that the procedures cause great pain. In the beginning, this is so. The manipulation of the muscle fascia is painful, but when the hands are removed the pain subsides.

An adjunct to Rolfing, involving a series of exercises that an individual who has been Rolfed can do at home, is called "structural patterning," and was developed by Judith Aston in association with Ida Rolf.

Ida Rolf's work is still actively offered by many practitioners throughout the U.S. and Europe. Training in Rolfing is available from the Rolf Institute of Structural Integration and others.

Further Resources

Ida Rolf wrote two books on the subject: *Rolfing: Reestablishing the Natural Alignment and Structural Integration of the Human Body for Vitality and Well-Being* and *Rolfing and Physical Reality*. Initially published as *The Bulletin of Structural Integration*, the journal devoted to Rolfing currently goes by the name *Structural Integration: The Journal of the Rolf Institute*. The Rolf Institute of Structural Integration is now located in Boulder, Colorado.

• •

140 Alexander technique

Exercises that enhance bodily awareness through the head-neck relationship.

The Alexander Technique is named after its developer and founder, F. Matthias Alexander. The technique provides a method of awareness training that enables the individual to experience the way his muscular and skeletal systems are used, both during movement and at rest. Once this becomes part of conscious awareness, an Alexander Technique teacher can then show the patient how to choose more appropriate ways to use their body.

The Alexander teacher helps the patient to come to this new awareness by a series of movements, exercises, and by the "laying on of hands." An example will illustrate this. You are with an Alexander Technique teacher, lying on your back on a massage table. The teacher softly but firmly places their hand under your neck and directs you to raise your right leg, bending it at the knee as you do so. When you raise your leg, you can feel the muscles in your neck tighten and contract against the teacher's hand, demonstrating how you use your neck muscles to "help" your leg muscles. If you can learn to become aware of this unnecessary neck tension, you can go on to learn how to correct it.

Further Resources

F.M. Alexander's writings have been collected by Edward Maisel under the title *The Resurrection of the Body.* The American Alexander Center is located in New York. An article, "The Alexander Technique" by Ilana Rubenfeld and Edward Rosenfeld, appears in *Workshops of the Mind,* edited by Bernard Aaronson.

· ·

141 Autogenic training
Speak to your body.

Autogenic training, also known as autogenic therapy, was developed by J. H. Schultz. Autogenic training is a combination of psychotherapy and psychophysiological exercises. The emphasis is on combining mental and physical functioning.

Autogenic training includes two sets of exercises, standard and meditative. The six standard exercises are to be executed in a quiet place, with low lights, loose clothing, in either a sitting, reclining, or horizontal position, with the eyes closed.

The first standard exercise is designed to affect the neuromuscular system. Key phrases can be said out loud or just thought about subvocally. A key formula is "My right (left) arm is heavy." The heaviness is indicative of true relaxation. The second exercise deals with the vasomotor system. The formula is "My arm is warm." This can cause the expansion of blood vessels in the desired area. The third exercise deals with the heart. The key formula is "Heart beat calm and regular." The fourth exercise concerns the respiratory system. The key formula is "It breathes me." This can produce relaxed, natural breathing. The fifth exercise applies to the central nervous system. The key formula is "My solar plexus is warm." This can bring calming. The sixth exercise concerns the cranial region. The key formula is "My forehead is cool."

These exercises are to be attended to with *passive*, rather than intensive or fixed, concentration. When first doing the exercises, thirty seconds to a minute is sufficient. After several months, the time can be extended to over a half hour.

The meditative exercises are for advanced autogenic students. The therapist usually tests to be sure that the standard exercises can be maintained without effort for more than a half hour.

The meditative exercises are tried and practiced over a period of months. The patient meditates on:

spontaneous phenomena (whatever arises in the mind)

spontaneous colors (envisioned without prompting)

colors at will (intentionally thinking of red, yellow, etc.)

imaginative objects (again, whatever emerges in the mind)

imaginative abstracts (freedom, truth, etc.)

feelings (emotions)

interrogations of the unconscious

Further Resources

J. Schultz and W. Luthe have already published two standard texts: *Autogenic Training* and *Autogenic Therapy*. Further information and a summary of the work is included in Luthe's article in the Charles Tart book *Altered States of Consciousness*. The article and the books give references for further reading. A review of some of the exercises is included in R. S. de Ropp's *The Master Game*.

. . . .

142 Flagellation

A post-sauna session with branches can change blood flow and get you high.

When the body is beaten, the histamine content in the bloodstream sky-rockets and one can get very high despite being hurt. Excessive beating is quite dangerous, of course.

Flagellation in a positive sense is used in steam baths, sweat lodges, and saunas to stimulate the circulation of the bather. After one is in the steam bath or sweat lodge for some time, the intense heat expands the skin and opens the pores. At this point it is best to flagellate the skin, usually with soft, leafy oak branches, in order to bring more blood toward the surface. This change in the circulation of blood helps the cleansing of the pores and brings about a tingling feeling in the skin. Some people have reported feelings of being high because of the change in blood flow brought on by a combination of heat and flagellation.

. . . .

143 Hypnosis

A state of unawareness.

Self-hypnosis is mentioned in No. 19, where instruction is given on hypnotic induction. However, many professionally trained hypnotists hypnotize others for purposes of relaxation, psychotherapy, restoration and cure, psychic exploration and experience, and for such frontier investigations as time distortion.

Ronald Schor defines hypnosis as follows:

Hypnosis is a complex of two fundamental processes. The first is the construction of a special, temporary orientation to a small range of preoccupations and the second is the relative fading of the generalized reality-orientation into nonfunctional unawareness.

Hypnosis can be used to change color perception, spatial orientation, perception of locale, and experience of heat, and even to produce mystical states. Many subjects have achieved astounding results through the use of Aaronson's hypnotic induction of the void experience.

Further Resources

See the resources for No. 19. For another view, see T. X. Barber's *Hypnosis: A Scientific Approach* and *LSD, Marihuana, Yoga and Hypnosis*. Later work in hypnosis took place as cognitive behavioral therapy came into vogue, especially with practitioners like Albert Ellis and Joseph Wolpe. See *The Clinical Use of Hypnosis in Cognitive Behavior Therapy: A Practitioner's Casebook* by Robin A. Chapman.

· ·

144 Massage
The pleasure of touch.

Massage is the rubbing or kneading of the body. It helps to relax the muscles and generally stimulates circulation. As Marshall McLuhan points out in his book, *the medium is the massage*. A massage is a pleasure to give as well as to receive.

There are specific massage techniques, and many states license professional masseurs. Following are some general considerations prepared by Esalen's Bernie Gunther for the art of massage.

Ask the person to be massaged to take a hot bath or shower first; it will add to their pleasure. Use ⅔ cup vegetable oil and ⅓ cup baby oil, then add something that smells good, such as oil of clove or almond extract. Try to maintain continuous touch, if only softly. The person being massaged will help you discover specifically how to touch when rubbing. Always try to rub toward the heart.

Stroke in circles on the neck, and then down from the head. Stroke up and down the arms and around the shoulders. Stroke and knead up and down the legs and thighs. Stroke up the stomach and down the sides. Stroke up in circles, then down in circles on the back. Lift the head gently, and corkscrew the fingers and toes.

George Downing gives the following suggestions in his *Massage Book*:

Try stroking with the balls of the thumbs

moving the fingertips with deep pressure in tiny circles

kneading

raking

stroking with the heels of the hands

stroking with the undersides of closed fists

drumming with the fingertips

making large sweeps and circles with the undersides of the forearms

When you are being massaged, feel it. Don't talk—just be with the touch. When the massage is over, lie still and enjoy the sensations.

Further Resources

A textbook on the subject, with many illustrations, is Beard and Wood's *Massage: Principles and Techniques*. Also recommended: George Downing's *The Massage Book*.

· ·

145 Kinesics

Reading body language to better understand ourselves and others.

K inesics, also known as body language, is an elaborate attempt to read the way in which we arrange our bodies in response to the variety of situations and environments that we experience during our waking hours. The main work on body-motion communication and its meanings has been done by Ray L. Birdwhistell.

Birdwhistell has developed a notational system, which he calls kine-graphs, that divides the body into eight different sections:

1 total head

2 face

3 trunk and shoulders

4 shoulder, arm, and wrist

5 hand and finger activity

6 hip, upper leg, lower leg, and ankle

7 foot behavior

8 neck

To give an example of the descriptors of this system I will list the ten indicated positions for the neck:

1 anterior projection

2 posterior projection

3 right lateral projection

4 left lateral projection

5 neck tense

6 neck sag

7 swallowing

8 Adam's apple jump

9 neck twist right

10 neck twist left

When this system, or systems like it, are mastered, then the nonverbal systems that most Westerners are committed to using in all social contexts become real communications rather than hidden movements of dubious meaning.

The next time you are speaking with someone and you notice him moving away from you, crossing his legs, folding his arms over his chest, and generally retreating, examine what you're saying that is driving him away.

Turning such awareness back on one's self is far more difficult, but can yield interesting and transformative results. As you are listening to someone pontificate on some subject, are your legs tightly crossed and your arms stretched across your chest? Are you holding your jaw tightly clenched? How's your breathing? Can you direct your awareness to your own body language? Doing so is often an illuminating exercise.

Further Resources

Ray Birdwhistell's work, *Kinesics and Context,* is scholarly and has an excellent bibliography. Julius Fast's *Body Language* is a popular presentation that lacks depth but reads easily. Some of the best material in this field can be found in Edward Hall's works, *The Silent Language* and *The Hidden Dimension.*

· ·

146 Laban movement

Writing body language.

Laban movement is based on the insights and work of Rudolf Laban, and is also known as Laban/Bartenieff Movement Analysis. Through awareness of inner states during movement, the subject can learn functional actions as well as emotionally expressive postures and gestures.

Laban developed a comprehensive system of notation for the positions of the human body. This system is often employed to "write" choreography, in much the way that music is written. Beyond delineating the individual positions of a dancer's body, it may be used to record an entire dance piece, including the complex interactions of any number of dancers dancing at the same time.

Laban notation can increase your awareness of how you use your body and what you experience during specific movements. In this sense the Laban system may become not only a map of movement, but of feeling.

Further Resources

Laban's work was carried on by his student Irmgard Bartenieff. The Laban/Bartenieff Institute of Movement Studies (limsonline.org) and the Dance Notation Bureau School (dancenotation.org) are both located in New York. Laban's book is called *The Mastery of Movement.*

147 Bates method

Eye exercises for rest and relaxation.

The Bates method, named after its developer, William Horatio Bates, is a system for improving vision so that glasses need not be worn. Unfortunately, after rigorous examination, it became clear that these exercises do not strengthen the eyes. While it's not recommended to use these techniques for improving your eyesight, they are helpful as a means to reeducate the process of seeing. When we see all things anew, our entire experience of life changes. As we change the quality of our sensory processing we change the quality of our consciousness.

One of these exercises is called "palming." The object is to provide rest and relaxation for the eyes by closing them. When the lids are closed, light can still penetrate. Bates suggests that the way to keep light from reaching the eyes is by placing the palms over the eyes, with the fingers being crossed on the forehead. This shuts out the light and allows the eyes to rest. The hands cover the eyes but do not touch them.

After resting the eyes, shift them from side to side and swing around, clockwise and counterclockwise. Do this with the eyes closed for about thirty seconds each. Palm the eyes before and after for rest and relaxation.

Another technique that Bates advocated was to look at a black surface so that one can see the black. This is also meant to be restful and relaxing to the eyes, especially when no attempt is made to see by holding or fixating. Just allow the black to calmly fill the field of vision.

Further Resources

The Bates book *The Bates Method for Better Eyesight Without Glasses* has been reissued after many years of being out of print. Aldous Huxley's long out-of-print *The Art of Seeing* describes the author's struggle with impending blindness and the use of the Bates techniques. There are many references to Bates and his method in the *Letters of Aldous Huxley*.

• •

148 Compressed time

Reprogramming your perception of time.

Compressed time has to do with investigations, now under way, that are examining the subjective experience of time. These experiments attempt to instruct and train individuals to manipulate, slow down, and speed up their experience of time.

Robert Masters and Jean Houston referred to their work in this area as accelerated mental process (AMP). They pointed out that we all experience AMP conditions: when we have a dream that seems to take hours and actually passes in seconds or minutes; during periods of emotional duress when one's whole life is experienced in a matter of seconds; and in other altered states of consciousness.

Masters and Houston used methods pioneered by Milton Erickson and Linn Cooper in hypnotic time-distortion. They induced a trance in their subjects and instructed them that they were then free to increase the amount of experience that would usually be possible during normal clock time. Their subjects included composers, dramatists, priests, and artists who returned from trance having had experiences of many hours, even days, in a matter of minutes.

In June 1969, Stewart Brand led a compressed-time workshop at the Esalen Institute. I quote the program description:

> Multiply time by $\frac{1}{12}$. An hour passes every 5 minutes. It's meal time every half-hour or so. Night is brief and oddly restful. Altogether it's an unboring, unhurried experience in which more (and different) accomplishments are possible than in normal time. The evening will be paced by clocks, sounds, lights, meals, and social cues to contain the events of a weekend.

This controlled environmental situation was uniquely effective. Brand said that people reported later that it had taken more than twenty-four hours after the workshop to adjust to normal clock time.

Using AMP techniques to alter our perception of time and duration can help us achieve simple altered states of consciousness. More recent research has verified earlier work in this field, see especially the review study of Ralf Buckley and other sources mentioned below.

Further Resources

The pioneering work in this field was done by Linn Cooper and Milton Erickson. Consult their book, *Time Distortion in Hypnosis.* Masters and Houston's *New Ways of Being, Mind Games,* and *Consciousness and Extraordinary Phenomena* also thoroughly explore the subject. Ralf Buckley's 2014 study, "Slow Time Perception Can Be Learned" (available at ncbi.nlm.nih.gov), provides a recent review of the literature in AMP. *Accelerated Expertise: Training for High Proficiency in a Complex World* by Robert R. Hoffman, Paul Ward, Paul J. Feltovich, Lia DiBello, Stephen M. Fiore, and Dee H. Andrews presents many of these themes from the perspective of business.

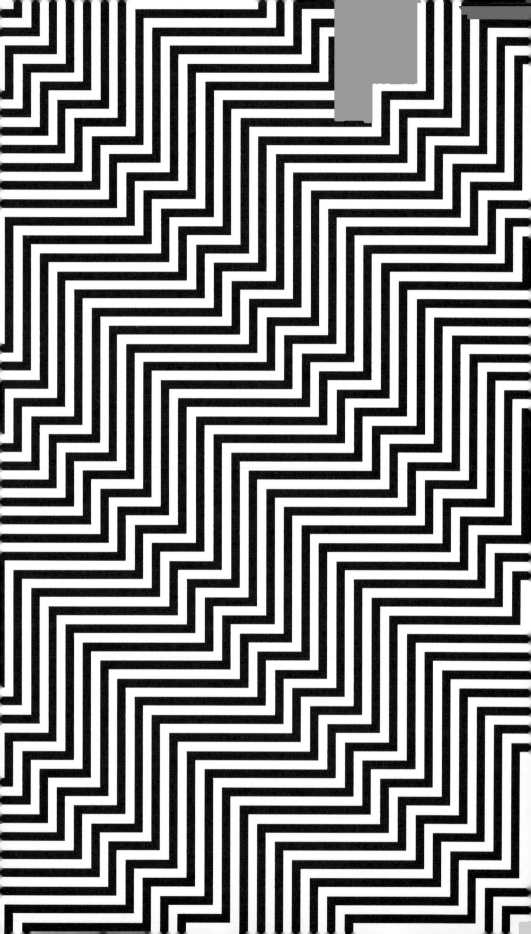

CHAPTER 7

RELIGIONS, MYSTICISM, AND MOVEMENTS

149 Yoga

It's not just postures.

Hindu religion, philosophy, and psychology are at the root of many developments that have reached the West in recent years. Hinduism brings man toward ultimate unity with the godhead, the Atman. Yoga is a *means* of achieving this unity.

If I were asked under what sky the human mind . . . has most deeply pondered over the greatest problems of life, and has found solution of some of them which well deserve the attention even of those who have studied Plato and Kant—I should point to India.
—HUSTON SMITH

There are many Yogas: Hatha, Vinyasa, Ashtanga, Bikram, Jnana, Bhakti, Karma, Raja, Mantra, Shiva, Swara. (Other forms of Yoga, including Agni, Kundalini, and Taoist will be discussed separately.)

Most popular Yoga forms are Hatha Yogas, the physical form known for its variety of postures (asanas). There is Jnana Yoga, which seeks knowledge of the godhead through intellectual knowledge; Bhakti Yoga, the Yoga of emotion, which seeks the godhead through the outpouring of love; Karma

Yoga, the Yoga of work, which is usually realized through either the path of knowledge (Jnana) or through the path of love (Bhakti); and Raja Yoga, which is the path of psychological experimentation. It is also here that one hears of the astounding physiological self-control accomplished by its practitioners. Such feats as walking on coals, sitting on nails, regulating body temperature in adverse climates, and live burial have been claimed by the Raja Yogi.

There are eight steps in the pursuit of Yoga. They are generally divided into *outer* and *inner* phases. They include:

1 Abstinences (nonviolence, truth, no theft, chastity, and nonpossession)

2 Observances (purity, contentment, austerity, self-development, and constant thought of divinity)

3 The postures, positions, or asanas (The asanas are based on the placement of bodily centers. There can be, according to Yogic teaching, $84 \times 1,000$ potential positions for the centers. The 84 fundamentals are often reduced to 21 major postures.)

4 Control of the breath (Pranayama)

5 Removing the mind from concern with external objects (Pratyahara)

6 Concentration (Dharana)

7 Contemplation (Dhyana)

8 Ecstasy, bliss, or identification (Samadhi)

Different teachers, or gurus, emphasize different combinations of the above for the attainment of unity.

Further Resources

Essential books for the study of Yoga and Hinduism include *The Upanishads*; *The Bhagavad-Gita*; W. T. DeBary's *Sources of Indian Tradition*; H. Zimmer's *Philosophies of India* and *Myths and Symbols in Indian Art and Civilization*; *Hindu Polytheism* and *Yoga: The Method of Re-Integration* by Alain Danielou; *Light on Yoga* by Iyengar; *Fundamentals of Yoga* by Ramamurti Mishra; Vithaldas's *The Yoga System of Health and Relief from Tension*; Ramacharaka's *Hatha Yoga* and *Raja Yoga*; and H. Chaudhuri's *Integral Yoga*. The Huston Smith quotation is from his book *The Religions of Man*.

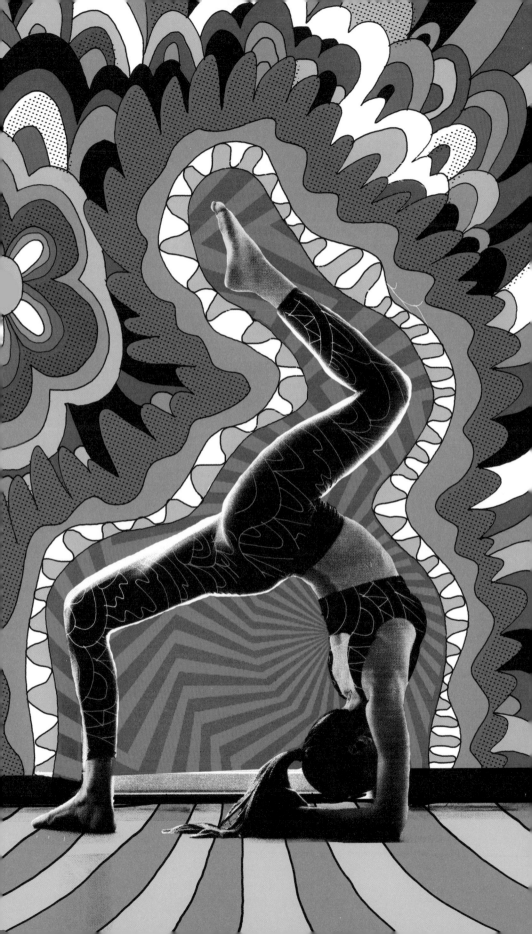

150 Transcendental Meditation

Concentrate on your mantra.

Transcendental Meditation, developed by Maharishi Mahesh Yogi and known to its followers as TM, claims to bring peace and happiness without struggle. The basic TM method involves assigning a personal mantra, or holy syllable, to the meditator. The meditator is instructed in simple meditation techniques and is told to sit in meditation, meditating on his mantra, forty minutes each day, twenty minutes in the morning and twenty minutes in the evening. It is better to sit before meals so that the body will not be busy with the digestive processes during the meditation period.

During these meditation periods, the focus is the personal mantra. Whenever one's attention wanders, the meditator gently brings their mind back to concentrate on their mantra. The aim is to develop a smooth, relaxed style of meditation.

There have been many claims for the effectiveness of TM. In this regard, a number of TM meditators have served as subjects for experiments that measured their brain-wave patterns, heartbeat, respiration rate, and other physiological indicators while they were practicing TM. While more research is still needed to determine the full extent of its effects on health, there are some promising results. In 2013, the American Heart Association released a statement saying that TM may be used to lower blood pressure. The American Psychological Association published a review of TM studies in 2012, concluding that the practice was beneficial for reducing anxiety and negative emotions, as well as for enhancing learning and self-realization.

Though some claims have been proven scientifically, others have proved dubious. After members of a prominent TM group said that TM had helped them learn how to levitate, that is, have their physical bodies leave the ground and hover in the air, doubts were cast on these claims. It was later revealed that the "levitators" were hopping and jumping off the ground and not levitating.

The movement has gained steadily in popularity. There are now TM groups in most major cities throughout the world. These groups maintain centers where interested individuals may be initiated into TM and given their personal mantra. The centers often have special rooms or areas set aside for meditation by TM members.

Further Resources

The *Science of Being and the Art of Living,* by Maharishi Mahesh Yogi, describes his personal development and the establishment of the TM movement. The TM movement is treated in a chapter of *The New Religions* by Jacob Needleman. The official TM website (tm.org) has links to contemporary studies of TM and its effectiveness. The filmmaker David Lynch, a practitioner and advocate of TM, runs a foundation focused on the practice (davidlynchfoundation.org) and wrote a book on his experiences titled *Catching the Big Fish: Meditation, Consciousness, and Creativity.*

• •

151 Agni Yoga
Freeing your cosmic energy.

Agni Yoga is fire Yoga, or fire union. There are two kinds of Agni Yoga now prevalent. One is the teaching brought back from the Himalayas by the Russian painter Nicholas Roerich and his wife. The Roerichs investigated central Asia, particularly Tibet and the Himalayan mountains. From this journey came their interpretation of Agni Yoga based on the Buddha of the future, Maitreya. The Roerich version of Agni Yoga draws on a variety of teachings present in the Vedantic schools of Hinduism and in the Mahayana Buddhist sects.

Their practice consists of paying special attention to diet, which they call astrochemistry, and meditation, to bring about the calm that eases the strains of reincarnation.

In the 1970s, Ralph Metzner and others called attention to another Agni Yoga teaching known as "actualism." This teaching was related to the initial works of Madame Blavatsky, Alice Bailey, and Maurice Nicoll. It centered around the work and experimentation of Russell Paul Schofield. Actualism purports to present the actual design of man as a cosmic being. It differs from other systems in that it aims to make the unconscious conscious by means of new methods that, according to Metzner:

> . . . eliminate the images and mechanisms obstructing and
> deviating energy flow through the various structures and
> functions of the personality systems.

Actualism posits three kinds of food: physical food, including the solids and liquids and gases that we eat, drink, and breathe; psychological food, including perceptions, feelings, thoughts, and attitudes; and energy food, which comes from life—light-channeled energy. Actualism's third law of energy states: "Obstructions to energy flow cause discomfort, if mild, or pain and 'dis-ease,' if strong."

The exercises of actualism are based on the principle that the individual will think, allow, and observe. An energy exercise involves thinking about a point of white light located some six inches above the center of the head. Once recognized through thinking, allowing, and observing, the light is thought of as opening up and pouring a shower of white-light energy over the entire body. It is advised that this exercise be done every day for a few minutes. Another use of this exercise is to focus the white light on the points in the body-energy system where blockage is experienced. These exercises are all done while sitting comfortably, straight-backed, in a chair, legs uncrossed, feet flat on the ground, hands on legs. A variation is to assume this position but place the right palm over the solar plexus and the left palm over the heart. While in this position the white-light exercises are repeated.

Further Resources

A series of Agni Yoga books are available through the Agni Yoga Society (agniyoga.org). These include most of the works written by Helena Roerich. The work of Russell Paul Schofield is reviewed, as is actualism in general, in Ralph Metzner's *Maps of Consciousness*. Schofield's poetry has been published under the title *Imprint Unmistakable*.

152 Tibetan Buddhism

Reaching spiritual and psychic heights through meditation, visualizations, and exercises.

When one talks about Tibet, one thinks not only of the country but of a state of mind, a mysticism generated by both the physical and the psychic heights. A number of Tibetan religious and mystical teachers called "tulkus" have settled in the West. The teachings they bring with them are arduous and thorough. There are five major schools of Tibetan Buddhism: Nyingma, Kagyu, Sakya, Gelug, and Gonang.

Tibetan Buddhist philosophy is based on compassion and the accumulation of merit. In order to accumulate merit the initiate works on the Bhumnda, or the exercise of 100,000. This is a series of exercises or meditations; each must be performed 100,000 times. There are five such exercises, the first of which is a prostration.

The hands are held with the palms close together but not touching. Holding the hands this way, they are then raised over the head, brought down in front of the throat, and then in front of the heart. The prostration is completed by touching the ground, with five simultaneous points of contact: the palms, the knees, and the forehead. While this bow is being executed, a series of complex concentrations as well as an involved visualization and the repetition of a mantra is also being executed.

The Tibetan initiate will complete 100,000 of these bows in one month's time. When studying in the West with émigré Tibetan masters, up to three months is usually allotted for completion of this, the first bhumi. The second bhumi is a series of 100,000 visualizations. The third bhumi is the recitation of the One-Hundred-Syllable Mantra 100,000 times, as part of a meditation procedure. The fourth bhumi is the visualization of the mandala of the entire universe in miniature. The fifth bhumi is the recitation of the meditation of the Universe. After this, the initiate meditates for three years, three months, and three days.

It was in Tibet that Tantric study came to its flowering. The tantras teach that there are seven energy systems in the body. These systems, or centers, are known as *chakras* (*cakras*). Chakra means "wheel." There are seven such centers postulated:

1 The root chakra, muladhara, at the base of the spine

2 The spleen chakra, svadhishthana

3 The naval or umbilical chakra, mani pura, at the navel or over the solar plexus

4 The heart chakra, anahata

5 The throat or laryngeal chakra, vishuddha, located at the front of the throat

6 The frontal or brow chakra, ajna, located just above and between the eyebrows

7 The crown chakra, or the thousand-petaled lotus, sahasrara, located on the top of the head

The Kundalini is thought of as a serpent (called by Art Kleps "an electric boa constrictor") that lies coiled at the root chakra. In meditation it begins to uncoil, releasing the energy of each chakra center as it ascends through the body. This is the origin of Kundalini Yoga, a practice for releasing kundalini energy through meditation, chanting, and yoga poses.

Further Resources

Jacob Needleman's *The New Religions* has a very good chapter titled "Tibet in America." The anthropologist Colin M. Turnbull has written, with Thubten Jigme Norbu, an excellent guide to the country. W. Y. Evans-Wentz's great works are all essential. Other fine books include Chögyam Trungpa's *Born in Tibet* and *Meditation in Action; Peaks and Lamas* by Marco Pallis; *Initiations and Initiates in Tibet* by Alexandra David-Néel; Herbert Günther's *Tibetan Buddhism without Mystification*; and Lama Anagarika Govinda's *Foundations of Tibetan Mysticism.* Books on Tantric Buddhism include the works of Sir John Woodroffe (pen name: Arthur Avalon); *Introduction to Tantric Buddhism* by John Blofeld; A. Bharati's *The Tantric Tradition*; C. W. Leadbeater's monograph *The Chakras*; and Omar Garrison's *Tantra: The Yoga of Sex.* Tibetan Buddhist groups and monasteries exist throughout the United States.

· ·

153 Tantric sex

The yoga of releasing sexual energy.

Tantric sex is a form of yoga; the only yoga that deals with human sexuality. Tantric sex is a means for channeling the sexual energy that is manifested in every man and woman. The rituals and instructions that form the core of tantric sex seek to release that sexual energy through the use of physical techniques, prayers, mudras (gestures) and chanting mantras (holy syllables and words).

The most important of the physical techniques is the practice of controlled breathing. The tantric masters give their disciples careful instructions: The breath flowing through the right nostril is masculine, hot and electrical; the breath that flows through the left nostril is feminine, cool and magnetic. The disciples learn to control their breathing so that they can make their breath flow through either nostril at will.

A typical sexual ritual is the Panchatattva, or secret ritual. Usually this is performed by a husband and wife. To begin, the guru selects the proper mandala (a magical, circular meditation image) for the rite and this mandala is drawn on the floor where the ceremony is to take place. The guru also gives the man and woman specific mantras to recite, both silently and out loud. The ceremony takes place in the evening in a dark room with many ritual elements such as candles, glasses, decanters, trays, and incense. Small portions of meat, fish, rice, and seeds are set in readiness. Alcohol is sometimes served as a prelude but is not required. The man and woman take a ritual bath to cleanse and purify themselves physically and spiritually. The man enters the room, empties his lungs, and begins a breathing ritual to equalize the air in his body. Twelve times he inhales for a count of seven, holds the breath for a count of one, and exhales for a count of seven. On the thirteenth breath of the cycle he directs his energy to a spot between his phallus and his anus. As he holds his breath, he helps to stimulate this area by contracting the muscles of his sphincter, releasing energy throughout his body. During this energy release he concentrates and meditates on the cosmic union between cosmic consciousness and cosmic energy. After this breathing cycle is completed, the woman enters the room and the man chants several mantras. Then some of the food is eaten and several prayers are intoned.

At this time the two partners go to the bed. The woman disrobes and sits, upright, at the side of the bed. The man stands in front of her and admires her, while saying certain mantras, as specified by their guru. He touches her heart, head, eyes, throat, earlobes, breasts, arms, navel, thighs, knees, feet, and yoni (vagina). The man then disrobes and they lie on the bed together, the woman on her back, the man on his left side, facing her. He makes sure that his breath is emanating from his right nostril as she raises her legs and brings her knees to her chest. He moves his head and chest away, bringing his phallus in touch with her genitals. She then brings her legs down and he moves his right leg between her legs. He then enters her, but not deeply.

The partners then lie together, relaxed and motionless, for thirty-two minutes, visualizing the flow of energy between them. At some time during the last four minutes, a rush of energy occurs. In order to avoid ejaculation the man holds his breath, curls his tongue backward in his mouth, and tightens his anal sphincter. After the thirty-two minutes (providing the man has not ejaculated), the energy is reversed and flows inward rather than outward from the partners. A sense of relief and joy is usually experienced at this time. If the man does ejaculate before the energy reversal, the ceremony can be started again.

In the Eastern traditions of Tantric sex there is no orgasm, but many Westerners practice variations of the Tantric procedures that include orgasm. Usually this orgasm is of a different nature than is usually experienced in the West. This is a relaxed, open, and flowing orgasm. By relaxing rather than tensing at the moment of most intense pleasure the participants can discover an entirely new way to experience the sexual and loving union.

Further Resources

The most explicit description of Tantric sex can be found in Omar Garrison's *Tantra: The Yoga of Sex*. Other treatments are in the works of Sir John Woodroffe especially *The Serpent Power*. Another, more Western, treatment of this material is to be found in *Sex and Yoga* by Nancy Phelan and Michael Volin.

• •

154 Body chanting

Chanting into the chakras creates a feeling of tingling and light-headedness.

This technique is from Bernard Aaronson, who learned it from Shyam Bhatnager, Pran Nath, and Harish Johari. The chant that was used on me was very similar to the *Live Very Richly You Happy One* chant described in No. 24.

For the spinal chant, the procedure is to lie down on a flat surface on your stomach. Your head rests on the ground, arms at your sides. The person who is going to chant places his or her lips approximately one half to one inch over the base of your spine. There is a chant said for each chakra. (For details on the chakras and their locations, see No. 152.) The chanter chants for at least five minutes over each spinal chakra. The teachers and therapists who are adept at this practice say that they experience the moment when a chakra opens and becomes activated. This is their signal to move on up the spine to the next chakra. No chanting is done for the seventh chakra, at the crown of the head. The person whose spine has been chanted over should be encouraged to lie still for five or ten minutes after the chanting has ended. The vibrational effect on the spine and the body as a whole can last as long as three hours.*

In addition to spinal chants, there are frontal chants and full-body chants. When selecting places to chant over, remember that the vibrations will be releasing energy.

A most extraordinary method of body chanting is to have the one to be chanted on lie on either his back or stomach on top of some large speakers: The chanting sounds from the speakers will pass through the body.

The basic feeling of this vibration effect is tingling and lightheadedness. The body seems much looser, colors are brighter, and most sounds seem clearer. It's a feeling of "loose clarity."

Further Resources

See resources for No. 24.

155 Taoism

The Way.

Taoism is a way of thought derived mainly from the teachings of two Chinese masters, Lao-Tzu and Chuang Tzu. Academic arguments rage over whether the collected works that appear under these two names are from two minds or many. The answer is not important here.

Tao means "Way" (as well as many other things). It is the Way of Life, the Way of Truth. The major work attributed to Lao-Tzu is the *Tao Teh Ching*.

Traveling the Taoist way is a nonordinary reality, a special experience.

Once Chuang Chou dreamt he was a butterfly, a butterfly flitting and fluttering around, happy with himself and doing as he pleased. He didn't know he was Chuang Chou. Suddenly he woke up and there he was, solid and unmistakable Chuang Chou. But he didn't know if he was Chuang Chou who had dreamt he was a butterfly, or a butterfly dreaming he was Chuang Chou.
—FROM CHUANG TZU (BURTON WATSON'S TRANSLATION)

Bend and you will be whole.
Curl and you will be straight.
Keep empty and you will be filled.
Grow old and you will be renewed.
Have little and you will gain.
Have much and you will be confused.
Here is the Way of Heaven:
When you have done your work, retire!
—FROM LAO-TZU'S *TAO TEH CHING* (JOHN WU'S TRANSLATION)

Other Taoist texts that have survived aim at the liberation of consciousness through the control of breath, much like Hatha Yoga, and through the circulation of light in the practitioner, much like Agni Yoga.

Further Resources

The major texts of Taoism are the collected writings attributed to Lao-Tzu under the title *Tao Teh Ching*. The main translation is by Arthur Waley, *The Way and Its Power*. A good modern translation is by J. C. H. Wu, *Tao Teh Ching*. The works of *Chuang Tzu* are in a fine translation by Burton Watson. H. G. Creel's *What Is Taoism?*, H. Welch's *Taoism*, and S. Waley's section on Chuang Tzu in his *Three Ways of Thought in Ancient China* all make good commentary on the Way and its development.

Taoist alchemy is presented in the original forms in Lu K'uan Yu's (Charles Luk) *Taoist Yoga*. A less sexual treatment of material from a similar source is *The Secret of The Golden Flower,* translated and explained by Richard Wilhelm and with additional commentary by C. G. Jung. The *I Ching,* a basic Taoist text, is considered in No. 181.

• •

156 Confucianism

Where personal enlightenment meets social organization.

The works of Confucius, Mencius, and Hsün Tzu form the basis of the ancient Chinese way of social organization that is known as Confucianism.

The religion scholar and writer Huston Smith discussed Confucianism as a means of enlightenment. Commenting on possible means of planetary organization for the future, Smith suggests incorporating the essentially Western skill of utilizing technology, the essentially Eastern skill of investigating the Self and the self, and the essentially Chinese (Confucian) skill of organizing men into groups. He writes:

> I believe that the Confucian concept of jen, which translates literally as tribesmen, freemen, or equal men, is the one social concept that might find success in helping us orient ourselves toward planetary retribalization. In Confucius's time, jen stood for cultivating human relationships, developing interpersonal faculties and abilities, and upholding human rights, often requiring the sublimation of one's own personality. Confucius said: Jen should never be abandoned even though one goes off to live with the barbarians.

Further Resources

The essential works of Confucian thought have been gathered together by C. Chai and W. Chai under the title *The Humanist Way in Ancient China.* The *Analects of Confucius* have been translated by Arthur Waley. The works of Mencius have been translated by D. C. Lau, treated by Waley in his *Three Ways of Thought in Ancient China,* and analyzed for meaning by I. A. Richards in *Mencius on the Mind.* The *I Ching,* a basic Confucian text, is considered in No. 181. Ezra Pound's translation of the *Classic Anthology* has appeared under the title *The Confucian Odes.* Confucianism in China today is the subject of Paula Marantz's *American Scholar* article from 2012 (theamericanscholar.org).

157 Buddhism

To awaken, to know.

B uddhism as a religion, a philosophy, and a psychology comes from the historical character of the Buddha, Siddhartha Gautama of Sakyas, near Benares in India. The name "Buddha" means one who knows, one who is awake. Buddha woke up by sitting under the now famous bodhi tree and coming to his enlightenment. He formulated the Middle Way, a way between asceticism and indulgence.

Buddhism as a religion grew out of a background of Hinduism and was, in many ways, a rebellion against the Hindu practices of the time. Eventually, Buddhism divided into two sects, Hinayana and Mahayana, Lesser and Greater vehicles, little and big rafts. What follows is a discussion of the part of Mahayana Buddhism that seeks what the Buddha sought: to awaken, to know. That sect, which blends Indian dhyana (contemplation) practices with the Chinese Taoist Way, is known in China (where it began) as Ch'an and in Japan and most of the modern world as Zen Buddhism.

Zen is the essence of Christianity, of Buddhism, of culture, of all that is good in the daily life of ordinary people. But that does not mean that we are not going to smash it flat if we get the slightest opportunity.
—R. H. BLYTH

The main practice of Zen is dhyana or meditation, which in Zen is known by the Japanese word *zazen*, sitting.

Communication in Zen is through the koan (Japanese for the Chinese *kung-an*—general case, or case establishing some legal precedent). Koans are the records of the enlightenment of the masters. Koans are cases, records, or writings that illuminate by example or description.

D. T. Suzuki, who was almost single-handedly responsible for most of the interest in Zen in English-speaking countries, always enjoyed describing Zen with the Four Statements:

A special transmission outside the Scripture;
No dependence on words or letters;
Direct pointing at the Mind of man;
Seeing into one's Nature and the attainment of Buddhahood.

Huston Smith has observed:

A group of Zen masters, gathered for conversation, have
a great time declaring that there is no such thing as
Buddhism or Enlightenment or anything even remotely

resembling Nirvana. They set traps for one another
trying to trick someone into an assertion that might imply,
even remotely, that such words refer to the real things.
Artfully they always elude the shrewdly concealed traps
and pitfalls, whereupon the entire company bursts into
glorious, room-shaking laughter, for the merest hint that
these things exist would have revealed that they are not
the true masters of their doctrine.

Some koans:

Kui Cheng said: Do not try to conjecture about Buddha
Dharma [Truth] by employing this bodily mind of yours
Where can you start to put it into words? Is there a
Dharma to which you can draw near? from which you
can withdraw? Is there a Dharma which is the same as
you? that is different from you? Why are you creating all
these difficulties for yourself?

A monk asked Chao Chou: What is the mystery of mysteries?
Chao Chou asked: How long have you been in
the mystery? The monk answered: A long time. Chao
Chou responded: If you had not met me you probably
would have been killed by the mystery.

A monk asked Shih Pei: What is myself? Shih Pei replied:
What you do with yourself.

Often koans refer to Bodhidharma, a Buddhist monk, coming from the West
(India). Bodhidharma brought dhyana from India to China, where it took
root in Ch'an. The monk asking a master what the purpose of this journey
was, like all other monks' questions to masters in koans, is asking: What's
it all about?

A monk asked Ching Chu: What is the purpose of
Bodhidharma coming from the West? Chin Chu said:
A slab of stone in midair. The monk bowed and thanked
the Master. Ching Chu asked: Do you understand?
The monk replied: No. Ching Chu said: It is fortunate that you
do not understand. If you do, it will break your head.

A monk asked Chao Chou: Does the Master go to Hell?
Chao Chou replied: Yes. The monk asked: Why? Chao
Chou answered: If I don't, who is going to teach you?

A nun came to Chao Chou and asked about the secret
teaching. Chao Chou felt her vagina. The nun said: Does

the Master have this? Chao Chou said: I do not have this, but you have it.

A monk asked Chu Tun about the Tao. The Master said: Do you think that you differ from the others? If a person can realize this, he then is one who has attained the Tao. He should feel that there is nothing different between himself and others in all matters even as [ordinary as] wearing clothes and eating meals. He has no mind to deceive. If he says, "I've got it! I understand!" Don't have anything to do with him!

A monk asked Chih Chin: What is the continuous flow of eternal reality? Chih Chin replied: It is like a mirror that forever shines. The monk asked: Anything over and above that? Chih Chin responded: Break the mirror and come to see me.

And finally, here is Blyth again:

. . . Zen tells us that the world is saved as it is. The ordinary man is the Buddha, time is eternity, here is everywhere. But this is only "so" if we know it is so. In the history of Zen, each monk as he becomes enlightened gloats over it almost indecently, just as the Buddha himself did, but how about all the poor unenlightened chaps, or those who died five minutes before they became enlightened? No, No! The universe must suffer, in being what it is, and we must suffer with it. Above all, the universe is a paradox, and we must laugh with and at it.

Further Resources

A good introduction can be found in the book *Buddhism* by Christmas Humphreys. The basic text of Hinayana Buddhism is *The Dhammapada*, which has been translated by Irving Babbit. Some fundamental texts retell Ch'an and Zen koans (see No. 22). The transmission of Japanese Zen (and with it the Ch'an tradition) was accomplished largely by D. T. Suzuki. All of his works on Zen are excellent, especially *The Essentials of Zen Buddhism*, edited by Bernard Phillips. An excellent comprehensive anthology is Nancy Wilson Ross's *The World of Zen*. Two modern approaches to Zen are revealed in Philip Kapleau's *Three Pillars of Zen*. Shunryu Suzuki, better known as Suzuki-Roshi, published a book of his talks, *Zen Mind, Beginner's Mind*. The most joyful of all the Zen writers is R. H. Blyth. His *Zen in English Literature and Oriental Classics* is most fulfilling. His finest work on Zen was cut short by his death. In *Zen and Zen Classics*, the first three volumes treat the history of Zen and Ch'an with Blyth spirit; the fourth volume is a supreme rendering of the Mumonkan collection of koans, and the fifth volume is made up of essays.

· ·

158 Tea ceremony

Opening the mind and body through a ritual both rigid and serene.

The Tea ceremony, also known as *Cha-no-yu* in Japanese, is an expression of Buddhistic consciousness. There are very specific and rigid rules for the serving of tea. These regulations guide the setting, the building, the implements, the participants, the sequence of the ceremony, and the tea itself. To be spontaneous within this rigidity, to let perfection *happen* despite all these prescriptions—this is *Cha-no-yu.*

What is most outstanding about the tea ceremony is its serenity and its beauty. Beauty surrounds the teahouse, in the gardens and ponds. The architecture of the teahouse represents another kind of beauty. The lamp, the furnace to heat the tea, the board that is used to support the kettle stand, the kettle stand itself, the kettle, the kettle hanger, and the jars where the leaf tea is kept are all made by craftsmen and masters with the utmost care and aesthetic consideration.

All of this beauty has but one aim: to open the mind, the body, the senses.

Further Resources

Two classics exist on the art of tea. One, *The Book of Tea,* by Okakura Kakuzō, is an essay and an appreciation. The other, A. L. Sadler's *Cha-No-Yu,* is the most complete work in English on the Tea Ceremony.

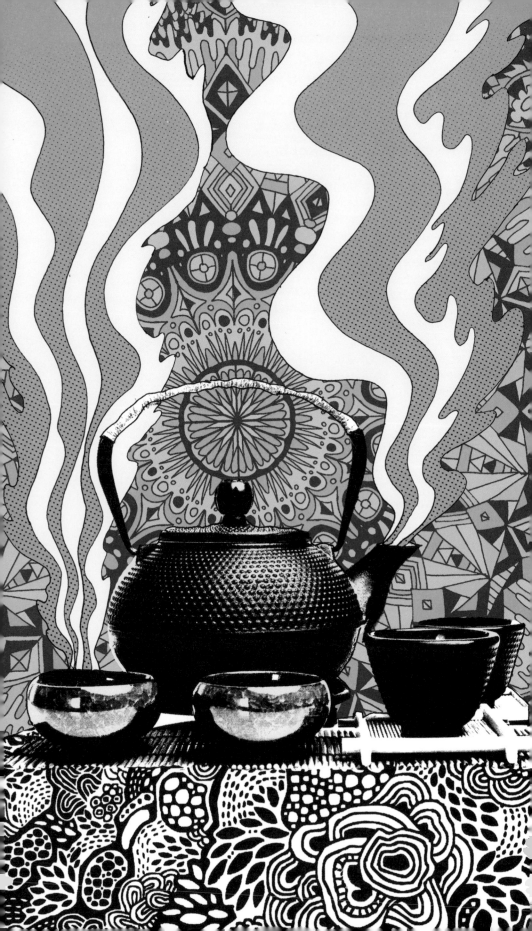

. . . .

159 Haiku

Seventeen syllables of beauty and brevity.

Haiku is a form of poetry that is written in seventeen syllables. Each poem contains a word that refers to the season described in the haiku. The following haiku are by the three greatest haiku poets of Japan. (All translations are by R. H. Blyth.)

Spreading a straw mat in the field
I sat and gazed
At the plum blossoms.
—BASHŌ

It is deep autumn;
My neighbour—
How does he live?
—BUSON

The autumn storm;
A prostitute shack,
At 24 cents a time.
—ISSA

Many Westerners have attempted to write haiku. Some have succeeded.

In a railroad yard,
bound for a world with flowers,
butterfly and I.
—JAMES HACKETT

In my medicine cabinet
the winter flies
died of old age.
—JACK KEROUAC

Further Resources

R. H. Blyth wrote the finest books on haiku in the English language. His two multivolumed works cover haiku and make it clear: *Haiku*, in four volumes: *Eastern Culture, Spring, Summer–Autumn, Autumn–Winter*; and *A History of Haiku*, in two volumes. Jack Kerouac's haiku were remembered by Allen Ginsberg in an interview published in *The Paris Review*, No. 37, Spring 1966.

160 Kendo and kyudo

The Zen arts of sword fighting and archery.

K endo is a Zen form of fighting with swords and sticks, while kyudo is a Zen form of archery. These are "artless" arts, effortless exercises. The aim is neither to defeat the opponent nor to strike the target, the target is the self, the swordsperson, the archer. Eugen Herrigel, a German philosophy professor who studied archery, described his master:

> He placed, or "nocked," an arrow on the string, drew the bow so far that I was afraid it would not stand up to the strain of embracing the All, and loosed the arrow. All this looked not only very beautiful but quite effortless.

The aim of kyudo and kendo practice is to become oneself. When wielding the stick or sword or loosing the arrow, only that activity will be taking place. In many ways kendo and kyudo are similar to the Zen meditative practice of sitting *zazen*. When one is a master of kendo and kyudo, the sword, the stick, the arrow, the bow, the target, the archer, the present moment, and the universe know no separation, no boundaries. All are one.

Further Resources

E ugen Herrigel's account of his bout with kyodo is in his *Zen in the Art of Archery* now published with another of his essays, *The Method of Zen*, in one volume titled *Zen*. Translator John Stevens's *Zen Bow, Zen Arrow: The Life and Teachings of Awa Kenzo* conveys the teachings of Herrigel's teacher, Kenzo.

161 T'ai chi ch'uan

Moving meditation.

T 'ai chi ch'uan is also known by the names Tai chi and Chinese boxing. It is moving meditation combining deep breathing with a series of slow movements in which the body weight is constantly shifting and the arms are describing circular arcs. Early development of T'ai chi ch'uan came from the

Taoist religious tradition. The contemporary form was codified by Chang San-feng in the twelfth century.

T'ai chi ch'uan looks like dancing but it is not. This appearance comes from the flowing way in which the exercises are executed. There are 37 basic exercises and postures called forms that are learned at the beginning of training. Then these basics are repeated with variations, bringing the total number of exercises to between 65 and 108, depending on the T'ai chi ch'uan master supervising the instruction.

The flowing exercises can be sped up into quick, sharply percussive movements. Springing from utter relaxation, these movements are particularly effective in combat because of the element of surprise.

Throughout T'ai chi ch'uan practice the emphasis is on centering the body, meditation, and relaxation. Later, the study of the *I Ching* may be undertaken to give philosophic dimension to the T'ai chi ch'uan practice.

Further Resources

Two good books on T'ai Chi Ch'uan are M. Cheng and R. W. Smith's *Tai Chi*, and Da Liu's *Tai Chi Chu'an and I Ching*; both are illustrated.

• •

162 Martial arts
Enlightenment techniques from the samurai.

Zen Buddhism was at the core of the samurai way of life in medieval Japan. From the samurai conditioning come a number of martial arts. All of them attempt to instill in the practitioner a way in which to gain their own enlightenment and peace.

Some of the most popular martial arts include judo (the art of balance and leverage), karate (unarmed striking blows), aikido (self-defense through becoming your opponent—no fighting or matches; only training), and *iaido*, (stick and sword use).

Further Resources

Judo and karate teachers abound. Watch your step. A good book on aikido is called *Aikido and the Dynamic Sphere*, by A. Westbrook and O. Ratti. See the United States Aikido Federation (usaikifed.com), the United States Judo Association (usja.net), and Shotokan Karate of America (ska .org) for a list of schools and resources.

163 Calligraphy and Sumie

Where writing and painting reveal the secrets of form and being.

Black ink fresh ground in water from an ink stick on a stone block, a flexible pointed brush, and a fresh piece of silk or rice paper are the only necessities. But these simple tools, in the hands of countless generations of artist-scholar-poet-philosophers in the East, have revealed the secrets of form and being.

Calligraphy as an art and a way of altering consciousness comes through aesthetic awareness, discipline, and the control of the breath. Each configuration is executed in a long, regulated exhalation of breath so that the flow is uninterrupted. Students are required to study and then copy the widely differing calligraphy masters. Once their talents are developed, they can begin to work on their own.

Each Chinese character, though a single unit, is made up of diverse parts in an asymmetrical arrangement. The way of seeing that calligraphy requires is a type of meditation, particularly when applied to painting. The subject is conveyed through its essentials, in a balance of shape and emptiness, with brushstrokes of sufficient power to reveal its basic nature, its breath—as well as its contours.

The expressiveness of *Sumie* (the Japanese name for brush painting) and calligraphy are unparalleled. A master can delineate any form, any gradation with a minimum of strokes, and, by only a slight change in pressure on the brush, completely alter the quality of a line or area of tone. Any subject may be treated, from the smallest sparrow to a range of mountains beneath the moon. Through the still, concentrated mind of the calligrapher great spontaneity is expressed with a few deceptively simple motions of the hand and arm. It flows on the paper almost without being noticed. Nothing has time to get in the way.

Calligraphy masters have spent years learning how "just" to write, "just" to paint.

Further Resources

Examples of Sumie and calligraphy are on view in Y. Awakawa's *Zen Painting* and J. Fontein and M. Hickman's *Zen Painting and Calligraphy*. An excellent introduction and manual is C. Yee's *Chinese Calligraphy*.

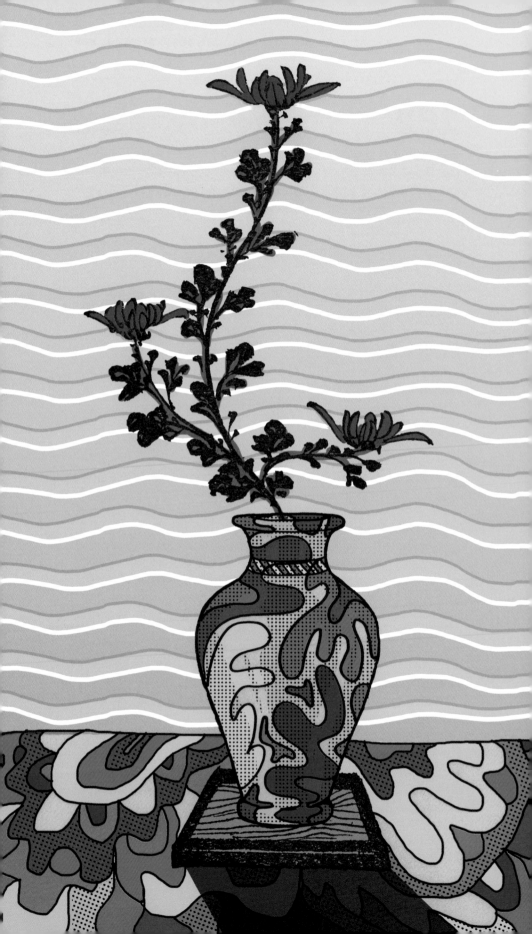

164 Flower arrangement

Beauty, simplicity, precision.

While Eugen Herrigel was studying the proper kyodo use of his bow and arrow, his wife was learning one of the ultimate Zen expressive forms: *ikebana*, or flower arrangement. Flower arrangement is much like the tea ceremony. There are many set ways and many prescriptions. The purpose is to let "you" shine through the flowers, to let the you who arranges be the flowers which are arranged. No difference—you-flowers.

Further Resources

Herrigel's *Zen and the Art of Flower Arrangement* is the classic treatment in English. There is information on flower arrangement in both Sadler's *Cha-No-Yu* and in Okakura's *The Book of Tea*. The former deals with flowers only in relation to the performance of the tea ceremony, while the latter treats the subject more generally. Ikebana International provides information on the practice on their website (ikebanahq.org).

165 Sufism

The wisdom of Islamic mysticism.

Sufism is the mystic tradition of Islam. The basis of Islam is the absoluteness, the One-ness of God. Allah is the One Lord and every man is His servant and creature. The prophets, including Muhammad, were sent merely to call man to Him.

The Sufi is the one who does what others do—when it is necessary. He is also one who does what others cannot do—when it is indicated.
—NURI MOJUNDI

Like the Zen and Ch'an masters and the Hasidim (see No. 22), the Sufis, or Qadiris, maintain a lineage of knowledge through reports on the actions, behavior, and sayings of their masters. Below are some Sufi tales:

> Bishr son of Harith was asked why he did not teach. "I have stopped teaching because I find that I have a desire to teach. If this compulsion passes, I shall teach of my own free will."

The candle is not there to illuminate itself.
—NAWAB JAN-FISHAN KHAN

When we are dead seek not our tomb in the earth, but find it in the hearts of men.
—*THE EPITAPH OF RUMI,* TRANSLATED BY IDRIES SHAH

Further Resources

The primary interpreter of Sufism in English is Idries Shah. The Koran is the basic work of Islam, and Sufism is part of the Islamic tradition. A readable translation is by Marmaduke Pickthall, under the title *The Meaning of the Glorious Koran.* Poetry by Haifiz, Rumi, and Attar (especially his *Parliament of the Birds* allegory) is fundamental to Sufi study. H. Corbin's massive *Creative Imagination in the Sufism of Ibn'Arabi* is difficult but worth the effort. D. M. Matheson's translation of *An Introduction to Sufi Doctrine,* R. Nicholson's *The Idea of Personality in Sufism,* and T. Burckhardt's translation of *Letters of a Sufi Master* are all good introductory texts. Modern Sufi thought is represented by the twelve-volume *The Sufi Message of Hazrat Inayat Khan.* Samuel Lewis was an initiate of Khan's and accepted by eight other Sufi orders. His *The Rejected Avatar* is a most unique tale.

· ·

166 Subud

Simple quiet communion with the divine.

Subud was founded by Mohammad Subuh. The center of Subud is a meeting, known as the *latihan,* which takes place twice a week and lasts for a half hour. People meet in gender-segregated rooms, and during the half hour no discussion or instruction takes place, no rules of conduct are enforced. The people at the latihan are free to do whatever they wish. They attend the latihan to submit to an acceptance of and receptivity to the power of God. Many who have attended latihans report remarkable experiences.

Further Resources

A good account of Subud is given, with references for further reading, in J. Needleman's *The New Religions*. There are three major books on Subud. One is a collection of talks by the founder, called *Subud in the World*. Another is Edward Van Hein's *What Is Subud?* The last is J. G. Bennett's *Concerning Subud*. Bennett was also part of the Gurdjieff-Ouspensky school and edited an interesting journal, *Systematics*. His two major works are *Energies* and *The Dramatic Universe* (4 volumes). The World Subud Association (subud.com) features recent developments in Subud.

• •

167 Jewish mysticism

Learning from Kabalist and Hasidic masters.

Jewish mysticism includes (especially) such groups as the Kabalists and the Hasidim. Much information is available on the *Bahir*, the first book of the Kabalists assembled in the twelfth century. The development of this group ranged from ascetic, monklike study to messianic movements.

Hasidism became prevalent in Eastern Europe in the eighteenth century. Martin Buber has collected many of the outstanding tales of the early and later Hasidic masters. The Zaddikim, the rabbis and wise men who are the subject of these tales, are identified by a variety of different names, which are standardized in the following stories:

> The Baal Shem said: "What does it mean when people say that Truth goes all over the world? It means that Truth is driven out of one place after another, and must wander on and on."

> One sabbath, a learned man who was a guest at Rabbi Barukh's table, said to him: "Now let us hear the teachings from you, rabbi. You speak so well!" "Rather than speak so well," said the grandson of the Baal Shem, "I should be stricken dumb."

> When the preacher Dov Baer realized that he had become known to the world, he begged God to tell him what sin of his had brought this guilt upon him.

Once when Rabbi Pinhas entered the House of Study, he saw that his disciples, who had been talking busily, stopped and started at his coming. He asked them: "What were you talking about?" "Rabbi," they said, "we were saying how afraid we are that the Evil Urge will pursue us." "Don't worry," he replied. "You have not gotten high enough for it to pursue you. For the time being, you are still pursuing it."

Before his death, Rabbi Zusya said: "In the coming world they will not ask me: 'Why were you not Moses?' They will ask me: 'Why were you not Zusya?'"

A community leader who was opposed to the rabbi of Kotzk sent him a message: "I am so great that I reach into the seventh firmament." The rabbi of Kotzk sent back his answer: "I am so small that all the seven firmaments rest upon me."

Further Resources

Buber's rendering of the Hasidic tales is referred to under further resources for No. 22. G. Scholem's *Major Trends in Jewish Mysticism* and E. Gewurz's *The Mysteries of the Kabalah* are good translations of Kabalistic thought. Elie Weisel retells many stories of the Hasidic masters in *Souls on Fire.*

· ·

168 Astrology
What's your sign?

Astrology is concerned with systematizing the relationships between the movements of heavenly bodies and events on earth. Its results can be evaluated by experiment and mathematical or statistical modes of investigation.

There are seven different types of astrology:

Natal: involving character development and personality based on the configuration of the zodiac, sun, moon, and planets at the moment of birth. These factors are also adjusted to the exact latitude and longitude at which birth took place.

National: concerning the developments of peoples, nations, and historical processes based on configurations similar to those used for individuals in natal astrology.

Horary: where questions are answered based on the time that the question was asked.

Astrometeorology: prediction of the effect of planetary influences on radio communication.

Medical: judging the nature and cause of illnesses and accidents, based on the relationship between the patient's birth configuration and the time of illness or accident.

Election: choosing the best person at the best time and place for specific chores or duties. Especially for people who have to work together, as on jobs in industry or crews of airplanes.

Ontological: the use of all of the above to investigate philosophical and psychological relationships.

The astrologer begins by looking up in standardized reference books the positions of the planets, luminaries, and constellations at a definite instant of time (the moment of one's birth, in natal astrology). From this information they will then draw a map, known as a chart, which shows the positions of and relationships between the heavenly bodies.

In a natal chart, the map is divided into twelve sections, or houses. The time of birth determines what constellation or sign will be on the horizon, thus ruling the cusp or boundary of the first house. The other signs will fall accordingly over the other houses. The luminaries are then placed in their proper astronomical positions within the houses. Since each luminary of each house of the natal chart concerns different areas of human life, the interactions among luminaries (called aspects) and between luminaries, zodiacal signs, and the houses, mirror the development of the subject's personality and lifestyle.

The difficult task of drawing accurate conclusions from the chart's numerous positions and relationships is accomplished through the skill and sensitivity of the astrologer. They must combine their knowledge of the elements of the chart and its aspects with their insight into the person whose chart is at hand. The interpretation made by an accomplished astrologer delineates both important past events and future potentialities. The predictions are usually an indication of the positive and negative forces that will bear on the subject rather than forecasts of specific events.

The perspective astrology gives on the causes and nature of past, present, and future events can distinctly alter our consciousness.

Further Resources

A good introduction to the subject is Louis MacNeice's *Astrology*. C. G. Jung's essay "Synchronicity" in Jung and W. Pauli's *The Interpretation of Nature and the Psyche* discusses the scientific basis of astrology. A good introductory text is the *A to Z Horoscope Maker and Delineator* by L. George. For more advanced work, see the many volumes of Alan Leo. The finest contemporary astrologer/philosopher is Dane Rudhyar. See his *The Astrology of Personality* and *The Planetarization of Consciousness*. A book for casting quick horoscopes with surprising accuracy is Grant Lewi's *Heaven Knows What*.

169 Magick

A mysterious art.

R eal magick is always secret.

Further Resources

T o help you through the secrets read Colin Wilson's novel *The Sex Diary of Gerard Sorme*. His nonfiction book *The Occult* provides a look at contemporary magic and magicians. Also study the published work of the foremost magician of the twentieth century, Aleister Crowley. E. A. Wallis Budge's *Amulets and Talismans* and Paul Christian's *The History and Practice of Magic* provide good background reading. F. Bardon's *Initiation into Hermetics* and *The Use of Magickal Evocation* are for the more advanced student.

170 Alchemy

What is the Philosopher's Stone of human consciousness?

To the scientist the aim of alchemy seems only to be the transmutation of base metals into gold. Though some alchemists were concerned solely with this, many were serious and dedicated thinkers who used alchemical symbols and ideas to probe religious, philosophical, and psychological problems. The "gold" for these men was wisdom and the creation of the whole, unmarred man. As Carl Jung has shown, the alchemists' symbols and methods were directly related to the workings of the collective unconscious and the individual psyche:

> Investigation of alchemical symbolism, like a preoccupation with mythology, does not lead one away from life any more than a study of comparative anatomy leads away from the anatomy of the living man. On the contrary, alchemy affords us a veritable treasure-house of symbols, knowledge of which is extremely helpful for an understanding of neurotic and psychotic processes. This, in turn, enables us to apply the psychology of the unconscious to those regions in the history of the human mind that are concerned with symbolism.

It was through symbols that the alchemists expressed both their investigations of the elements making up human consciousness and the ways to integrate them effectively. The issues raised by alchemy are not dead. Some of our contemporaries consider psychedelic drugs to be this integrative principle, the philosopher's stone of the new alchemy, and various masters have used alchemical methods in their own theoretical formulations—Gurdjieff's "Table of Hydrogens," for instance, posited a description of the elements of *matter* involved in man's consciousness.

Further Resources

Two introductory books are available, both called *The Alchemists*. One is by F. S. Taylor and the other by M. Caron and S. Hutin. *Mysterium Coniunctionis,* Jung's difficult treatment of the discipline, is found in Volume 14 of his collected works. Ralph Metzner's *Maps of Consciousness* contains a chapter on alchemy. A compendium of contemporary artists influenced by alchemy can be found at Levity (levity.com/alchemy).

. . . .

171 Anthroposophy

Is it possible to study the spiritual realm?

A nthroposophy, literally "man's wisdom," was the name given to the work of the group that Rudolf Steiner formed in order to carry out scientific investigations of the spiritual realm. Steiner's was an incredibly able mind, producing singular works in many fields, including education, architecture, botany, and agriculture, and studies of such men as Goethe and Nietzsche.

Anthroposophy is Steiner's attempt to lay down a cosmic history and guide to the wisdom of the universe. It includes much of the knowledge that he gained through out-of-body experiences and astral projection.

Further Resources

D etails on Steiner, his life and work, and anthroposophy are available from the Anthroposophical Society (anthroposophy.org). Some recommended titles from the many volumes of Steiner's work are *Occult Science: An Outline; Theosophy: An Introduction*; and *Knowledge of the Higher Worlds and Its Attainment.*

. . . .

172 Arica

A unique blend of meditation and philosophical study.

A rica is a training program developed by Oscar Ichazo. The name Arica is taken from the town in Chile where Ichazo trained his first group. The training consists of a variety of exercises that Ichazo integrated from many religious and mystical traditions, both Eastern and Western. Most of the exercises are experienced in the form of meditations. The focus of the meditations ranges over vibration, movement, sound, philosophical theories, planetary and galactic systems, music, kath (the center of the body, usually placed at or near the navel), tantra, kundalini, and others.

Ichazo says that the aim of the training is to produce a state of consciousness he refers to as the Permanent 24. The number 24 refers to a state analogous to satori (in Zen Buddhism) or Samadhi (in the yogic disciplines).

Further Resources

chazo has never published in English. John Lilly described part of his experiences in Chile during the initial Arica training and some of the group exercises in his book *The Center of the Cyclone.* Current information on Arica can be found at arica.org.

173 Religious pilgrimage

The challenges and rewards of a spiritual journey.

If you know of the existence of a religious or philosophical master or teacher that you feel will be just right for you, and you go to that master or find the source of that teaching, this journey is a form of religious pilgrimage. Another form is that practiced by the wanderer; they may make most of their life a search for the right teaching, the right teacher, and the right time and place for learning. The journey, especially if arduous, makes the experience in the place or learning from the master, all the more intense.

There are currently several pilgrimage organizations that make the process easier for the masses. For example, Birthright Israel brings Jewish youth to their holy land at no cost. Whether or not these organized trips detract from the power of a hard-won journey remains to be seen.

Further Resources

Baba Ram Dass's *Be Here Now* gives his view of the religious pilgrimage. Other views include Hermann Hesse's *Journey to the East*. René Daumal's *Mount Analogue*, and the Sufi classic *The Parliament of the Birds* by Attar. Some pilgrimage destinations: Chimayó in Santa Fe, New Mexico; Lourdes in France; Naag Mandir in Fiji; Medjugorje in Bosnia; the Golden Temple, the Mata Vaishno Devi temple, and the four sites of Char Dham in India; Mount Kallash in Tibet; the Western Wall in Israel; Our Lady of Guadalupe Basilica in Mexico; the Madron Well in England; and, of course, Mecca in Saudi Arabia.

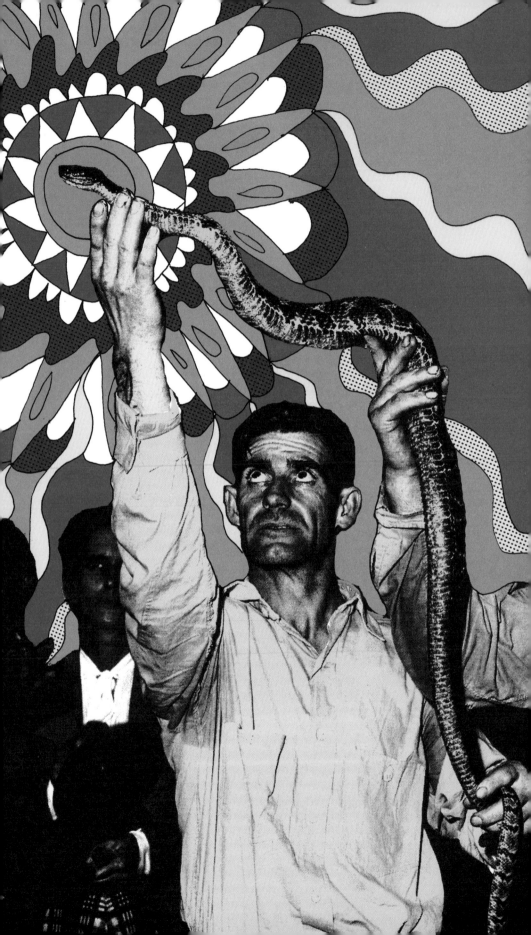

174 Revival meetings

Ecstasy, holy rolling, and other extreme states.

R evival meetings usually require a charismatic personality to bring them off. (See Faith healing, No. 177, and Charismatic speakers, No. 178.) But most people who attend them are already believers, and trances are usually the order of the day, or night. Faith healing, ecstatic movement, snake handling, and holy rolling are all instances of people experiencing extreme states of consciousness. If you become involved, it can happen to you, too.

Further Resources

T he resource material for No. 177 also applies here.

175 Religious conversion

An experience of transformation.

T o be converted, to be regenerated, to receive grace, to experience religion, to gain an assurance—there are so many phrases that denote the process, gradual or sudden, by which a self hitherto divided, and believed to be wrong, inferior, and unhappy, becomes unified and consciously right, superior, and happy, in consequence of its firmer hold upon religious realities. This at least is what conversion signifies in general terms, whether or not we believe that a direct divine operation is needed to bring such a moral change about.

The following excerpt, from William James's *The Varieties of Religious Experience*, written during the first year of the twentieth century, still best describes religious conversion. The process sweeps everything in its way, changes the Subject and transforms all that the Subject experiences. It is, of course, impossible to summon at will.

> What brings such changes about is the way in which emotional
> excitement alters. Things hot and vital to us today are cold
> tomorrow. It is as if seen from the hot parts of the field that the
> other parts appear to us, and from these hot parts personal desire

our dynamic energy, whereas the cold parts leave us indifferent and passive in proportion to their coldness. . . .

Now there may be great oscillation in the emotional interest, and the hot places may shift before one almost as rapidly as the sparks that run through burnt-up paper. Then we have the wavering and divided self. . . . Or the focus of excitement and heat, the point of view from which the aim is taken, may come to lie permanently within a certain system; and then, if the change be a religious one, we call it a conversion, especially if it be by crisis, or sudden. . . .

Neither an outside observer nor the Subject who undergoes the process can explain fully how particular experiences are able to change one's center of energy so decisively, or why they so often have to bide their hour to do so.

Further Resources

In addition to William James's thorough discussion in *The Varieties of Religious Experience*, material is available in George A. Coe's *Psychology of Religion*; C. Kirkpatrick's *Religion in Human Affairs*, and William Sargant's *Battle for the Mind*. Also see Anton Boisen's *The Exploration of the Inner World*.

• •

176 Séances
The practice of communicating with the dead.

Seances are meetings of people who wish to receive spiritual messages. Generally an attempt is made to communicate with the spirit of a deceased family member, friend, or acquaintance of someone at the séance. At other times, a séance might try to contact a spirit having to do with the power of an event or structure, such as a house.

Though often pictured as a scene in which everybody sits at a round table holding hands, séances occur more often with the participants standing or sitting in a circle with nothing inside the ring, except perhaps some symbolically significant object, like a crystal ball. The group dynamics of the situation, plus the intensive energies being produced, often combine to bring about altered states of consciousness.

The medium is the person who directs the activities at a séance. Many are women. A medium claims to have the power to contact spirits; usually these spirits are supposed to be aspects of human beings who are now dead.

A medium will usually attempt to make contact with the spirit and to have the spirit indicate its presence to the others taking part in the séance.

This demonstration is accomplished by some sort of unusual noise or movement in the séance room.

Many séances have been broken up when the medium has been exposed as a charlatan who uses tricks to imitate a spirit presence. There are many mediums in the United States, made particularly popular by television. It is up to you to decide if a medium's power is legitimate. Be diligent in your research before enlisting one for a séance.

177 Faith healing

When belief works miracles.

Physician, heal thyself! Patient, you may do the same. Though not all illness is caused by psychosomatic disorder, most are aggravated by a lack of understanding of the psychological conditions necessary for cure. The emotional environment developed by many faith healers is responsible for a great number of their successes. When the ill or lame patient knows that the healer they are to see has healed others, they feel it just might work for them, too. If the healer possesses enough personal or charismatic power it often *will* work. This concept is similar to that which enables positive thinking methods to be so effective for so many people. It all has to do with the way we live: If we think something is so, we tend to help it become so, sometimes even in the face of extraordinary hardship.

Further Resources

Westom LaBarre's *They Shall Take Up Serpents* deals with an unusual group in the southern United States. Coe's *The Psychology of Religion*, Sargant's *Battle for the Mind,* and Kirkpatrick's *Religion in Human Affairs* also discuss the subject.

178 Charismatic speakers

Greek *kharisma* = "divine gift."

Most of today's successful politicians are charismatic speakers. When they address the public, their method of delivery, their appearance, and their assumed social position vis-à-vis the group to whom they are speaking all combine to work a special kind of magic.

When you hear a speaker who can generate what seems like electricity, when everyone listening to them is caught up in the sound (not necessarily the content) of their words, then you are in the presence of a charismatic speaker. The next time you go to the political rally or a religious mass meeting, watch the crowd as you listen to the speaker. You'll see them nonconsciously lean forward, nod, bob in their seats, carry on subvocal dialogue, and grimace in reaction to things that aren't necessarily in the content of the words being spoken. You will be observing the special force of the charismatic speak upon their audience. Many people experienced President Barack Obama as a charismatic speaker; some consider President Donald Trump one, too.

179 Crowds

The danger and excitement when groups gather.

On a city street some eight or nine people have gathered to investigate an unknown and otherwise unnoticed phenomenon. As other people walk by, their eyes are drawn to the small group of people. Some walk over just to see what is going on. A crowd develops. The original group is standing huddled close together around a frantic man who is speaking rapidly and breathing in gasps. More people are streaming toward the crowd. The attraction is magnetic. People who are part of the crowd are pressed tightly against one another, straining to hear what is being said at the center. All of the people in the group are focused on the same spot; their sensory attention is concentrated on the crowd, their crowd.

Suddenly, someone breaks from the circle and runs down the street. Several people in the crowd give chase. Others stand and question each other in an attempt to orient themselves to the new events, to find out what's going on. People lose interest. They walk away. Others hang around, but there is no longer a center of activity; the focal point has disintegrated. The crowd breaks up.

In situations such as this, the consciousness involved is mass consciousness. Had the person who broke away failed to escape, there might have been assault, battery, or perhaps even homicide. Crowds have the power to affect these sudden, often senseless acts.

Further Resources

Elias Canetti's classic study *Crowds and Power* details all the altered states associated with groups. Also see Gustave Le Bon's *The Crowd* for an earlier study of the same phenomenon.

• •

180 Spontaneous gatherings, flash mobs, and happenings
Random acts of exuberance.

In 1956 and 1957, the artist Allan Kaprow chose the term "happenings" in order to describe what has come to be known as sometimes spontaneous performance art (the Beat generation novelist and poet Jack Kerouac called Kaprow "The Happenings Man"). Happenings became a general term for so many different kinds of artistic events. Whether they were planned or totally spontaneous, happenings were events to experience. Mayhem, junk, a stage, crowds, paint, actors and actresses, an audience, sets, all out of the familiar, calm surroundings; all removed from the normal.

Over the decades, happenings molted into flash mobs and other varieties of spontaneous gatherings. Flash mobs came into their own at the same time that YouTube videos spread content to billions. So when, suddenly, large groups of musicians and/or singers and/or clowns and/or people in other kinds of costumes and garb all converged on a public location to play music, sing songs, do acrobatics, and perform so many other feats of wonder, the flash mob became unexpected entertainment, joy, and sometimes bewilderment to many.

Further Resources

A search for flash mob stories and videos will bring up thousands of examples. YouTube is a primary source for these videos. A broader, more philosophical view can be found in *Smart Mobs: The Next Social Revolution* by Howard Rheingold. Event websites like meetup.com are good places to look for a flash mob event near you.

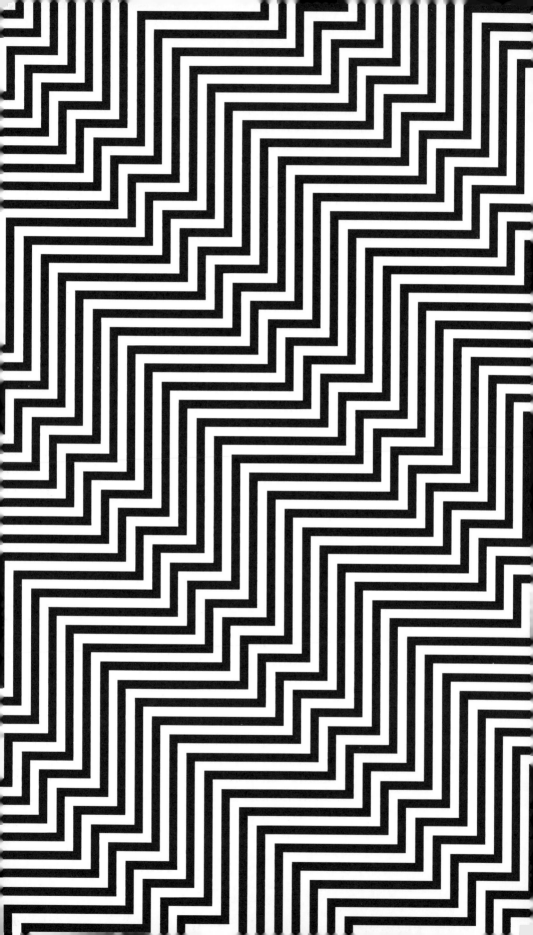

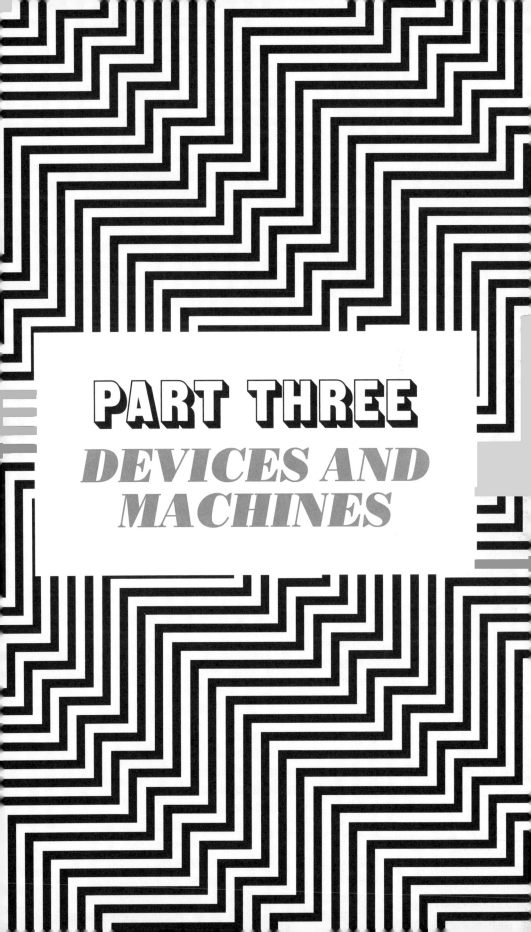

PART THREE

DEVICES AND MACHINES

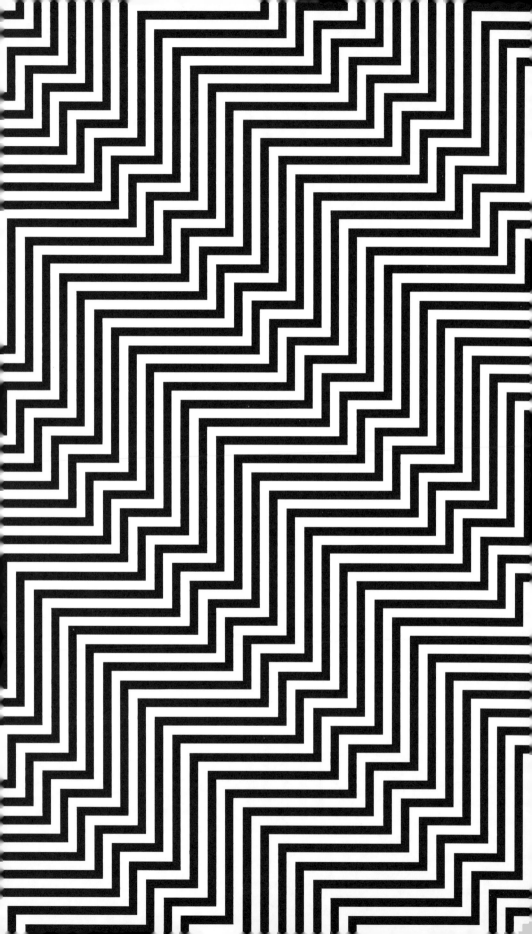

CHAPTER 8
NONELECTRIC

- -

181 *I Ching*

A text that operates as oracle and philosophical guide.

The *I Ching* or *Book of Changes*, now the most important of the five classics of Confucianism, came to life as an oracular work more than three thousand years ago. Its core is a series of sixty-four symbolic figures called hexagrams, each of which is one of the possible combinations of six broken and/or unbroken parallel lines. Broken lines stand for yin, the dark, feminine, receptive, negative principle; unbroken lines stand for yang, the light, masculine, creative, positive principle. Each hexagram is an aspect of life or a life situation. Each line shows a different aspect of the situation pictured by the hexagram. Associated with each hexagram are commentaries which expound on its meaning. The most extensive of which was written by Confucius and his pupils.

As an oracle, the book may be consulted with either coins or stalks. Keeping the question constantly in mind, you cast the coins or stalks in a prescribed manner and, from the resulting configuration of unbroken and broken lines, find your hexagram. In most instances, some lines are changing lines leading to a second hexagram.

The power of oracular devices, like the *I Ching* and Tarot card reading (No. 182), to alter consciousness has been known for millennia. These methods allow us to draw back the curtain from the future: the unknown, even the unknowable. They change us by inducing us to focus on our futures and our fates, on the things in life that require nothing but surrender.

Years ago, when we had just purchased a new house, my then wife and I decided we should consult the *I Ching* to see what that oracular book would tell us about what this new home would mean for us, as a couple, in the future. I no longer remember the first hexagram that presented itself to us, but I remember vividly what that initial hexagram's lines changed into: the hexagram configuration called "Breaking Apart." My wife ran from the room crying, and I was devastated by the prognostication. As predicted, within several years, we agreed to divorce, though we remain very good friends to this day.

Carl Jung considered the *I Ching* to be based on as valid an experimental method of investigation as Western science. He called the principle involved *synchronicity*, which means the occurrence at the same time of two events which, though unconnected by cause and effect, are nonetheless related.

Including information on government, numerology, astrology, cosmology, meditation, and military strategy, the *I Ching* transcends its divinatory function to become a philosophical guide to Chinese thought, both Confucian and Taoist.

When Jung consulted it regarding itself, it gave the hexagram *ting*, the cauldron, for which the judgment is "Supreme good fortune. Success."

This reflects the basic concept of the *I Ching*—that nothing in life remains static—all is impermanent—all is ever-changing.

Further Resources

The most popular edition is the Baynes rendering of Richard Wilhelm's transliteration. This work is very usable but makes the *I Ching* seem more romantic, less gutsy than it really is. Pay attention to the boldface type: the image, the judgment, etc. Wilhelm's son, Hellmut, has provided the best introduction in his *Change: 8 Lectures on the I Ching.* This book should be read before consulting the real thing. Spend time also with volume 2 of Joseph Needham's monumental *Science and Civilization in China: History of Scientific Thought.*

• •

182 Tarot
Cards that awaken future consciousness.

The Tarot is another oracular device in the form of a deck of cards. Though its exact origin is not known, those who connect the Tarot with Hermetic philosophy and occultism trace the inception of its symbolism back to dynastic Egypt. Similar theories point to the fact that the cards were often used for gambling, which was the intention of the formulators of the Tarot system. Used in that way, even those unappreciative of occult significance would have use for the deck of metal or leather cards known as the Tarot.

The deck of cards now used for the Tarot are paper and divided into two sections, known as the Major and the Minor Arcana. There are twenty-two cards in the Major Arcana and fifty-six (sometimes fifty-two) in the Minor Arcana. The Minor Arcana is like the contemporary deck of cards. This means the Minor Arcana has four kings, queens, knights, and knaves (the knight does not appear in regular card decks—thus the fifty-six cards in the Minor Arcana), as well as aces, deuces, and so on up to ten. The four modern suits known as hearts, diamonds, spades, and clubs, are, in the Tarot, pentacles or money, cups, swords, and wands.

The twenty-two cards of the Major Arcana bear the following pictures and symbols:

1 Magician	9 Hermit	16 Tower Struck by Lightning
2 High Priestess	10 Wheel of Fortune	17 Star
3 Empress	11 Strength	18 Moon
4 Emperor	12 Hanged Man	19 Sun
5 Pope	13 Death	20 Judgment
6 Lovers	14 Temperance	21 Fool
7 Chariot	15 Devil	22 World*
8 Justice		

The Tarot has been described as a philosophical machine, an instrument of cognition, and the algebra of occultism. It is all of these, to be certain, and more. The methods of distributing the cards properly depends on the teacher. Some use only the Major Arcana, some only the Minor Arcana, some both.

The various images of the Major Arcana are thought to be highly charged, archetypal symbols carrying a power that has been vested in them over centuries of use. By correctly reading the placement and appearance of the cards, many claim to be able to describe events that have already transpired as well as gain impressions of events that will occur in the future. Psychologist and consciousness researcher Ralph Metzner suggests using the images of the Tarot as a form of guided fantasy to see what kinds of associations come from the pictures on the cards. Pick out a card that has particularly positive associations for you and tack it to the wall. Live with the card and see what it guides you toward.

*In some systems, 21 is the World and 22 the Fool, but when that is the case the Fool bears no number, or is known as the zero card.

Further Resources

The most popular book on the Tarot is A. Waite's *The Pictorial Key to the Tarot*. Other useful works include M. Sadhu's *The Tarot;* G. Moakley's iconography and history, *The Tarot Cards;* and E. Gray's *A Complete Guide to the Tarot*. There are three interesting decks available. The standard is the deck designed by Waite and Colman. Two other decks include the Palladini deck from the East Coast, and the New Tarot for the Aquarian Age from California. *Maps of Consciousness* by Ralph Metzner has an explanatory chapter on the Tarot that is most informative.

• •

183 The ten oxherding pictures

The path to enlightenment, in ten pictures.

The Ch'an and Zen Buddhists have a teaching technique designed to help anyone on the path to enlightenment, also known as *satori* and *kensho*. Enlightenment is the ultimate goal of Zen, to live fully, in the now.

But such a journey is a slippery slope. As one Zen proverb notes: Before I knew anything of enlightenment, mountains were mountains, trees were trees. After I learned a little about the path to enlightenment, mountains were no longer *just* mountains, trees no longer *just* trees. But once I attained *kensho*, mountains were, once again, *just* mountains, trees *just* trees. Or, more prosaically: Before *satori*, chop wood, carry water, after *satori*: chop wood, carry water.

One of Ch'an and Zen's most illuminating teaching techniques about the path to finding the self and full realization are the ten oxherding pictures. Each picture shows a way station on the path to *kensho* with the seeker searching for the self, here symbolized by the ox.

The first picture shows the man searching for the ox. The second picture shows the searcher finding traces of the ox. The third picture shows the man finding the ox; and, in the fourth picture, catching the ox. In the fifth picture, the man tames the ox, while in the sixth picture the man returns home riding on the back of the ox. In the seventh picture, the ox is forgotten, but the man remains. In the eighth picture, there is nothing, neither ox nor man; and, in the ninth picture, the world reappears, but, as always, all things are changing. In the tenth and final picture, the man reappears, with open hands, and is in the marketplace, face to face with another man.

Further Resources

There are many versions of the ten oxherding pictures. *The Ox and His Herdsman: A Chinese Zen Text* has commentary by Master Otsu (English translation by M. H. Trevor).

· ·

184 *Finnegans Wake*

You know, LSD is the lazy man's Finnegans Wake.
—MARSHALL MCLUHAN TO TIMOTHY LEARY

To many would-be readers, James Joyce's monumental opus is unreachable. For a select few who have discovered a simple method of entry, the book is a revelation of major cultural significance. The key is that the book is an oral record. It is meant not only to be read, but to be read out loud, to be shouted, to be sung, to be laughed; to be laughed at and to be laughed with and to be laughed through. In order to be known, *Finnegans Wake* must be heard. Speak the words out loud. The book will come to life.

Eric McLuhan prepared one of a number of guides through this most fantastic work of words of the twentieth century. Many of the notes below are from his book *The Role of Thunder in Finnegans Wake*.

Finnegans Wake is an account of the social dynamics and interplay of technology and culture in a variety of historical configurations. It is constructed as a total environment where the varieties of relationships described are expressed as resonance. A conscious awareness of the separate and interlocking sensory modalities is stressed. Joyce wanted the reader to approach the work with both visual and auditory perceptiveness, simultaneously. In addition, various evocations of space reach out for our tactile sense and consideration.

These are the words the reader will see, but not those he will hear.
—JAMES JOYCE, IN A LETTER DESCRIBING THE *WAKE*.

The metaphors and puns in the *Wake* attempt to liberate our linear modes of thought, reinforced by years of visual, nontactile, nonauditory cultural indoctrination. Much of the characterization in the *Wake* describes the world changes and fluctuations between linear and nonlinear forms of information processing brought about by media transformations.

Two parts of the *Wake*'s construction make this clear: the five major characters: HCE, ALP, Shaun, Shem, and Izzy; and the ten thunderclaps, each of one hundred letters. These thunders are multilayered word compounds. They can be divided into three sections. The first section, the first

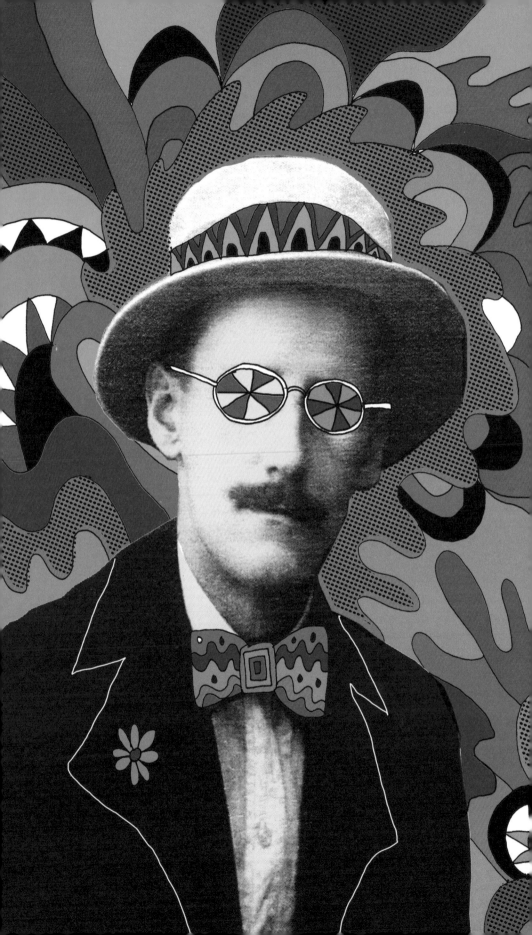

three thunders, describes the detribalization of mankind through industrialization and the introduction of linear media. The second section, the fourth through sixth thunders, describe the totality of the civilizing processes that take place with industrialization. The last section, thunders seven through ten, describe what Joyce could see (the book was completed in 1939) of the coming eventual retribalization at the hands of the new world-surrounding electric technologies and media.

The characters play out this history and future in the following representations. HCE is everyman, detribalized, civilized, industrialized, our public, us. ALP is the woman behind the man (HCE) and the technological environment that helps to make the man what he is, often without his total awareness of the process. Izzy is her helper, sometimes only by manifestation, who stands for the rising portions of environmental powers of transformation. The sons of HCE, Shaun and Shem, are the polarities of cultural transformation. Shaun, the bureaucrat, always needs the present/future orientation of Shem, the artist, to help move out of the past's status quo.

As these characters play out our future destinies, the thunder intercedes at the moment of peak intensity, bringing at first fragmentation, as in environmental metamorphosis, and eventually reunification of the human sensorium.

Joyce noted that he was writing the Wake *deliberately "after the style of" television—that is, his style is one that uses simultaneous and inclusive forms of awareness and extends to multiple-leveled patterns recognition.*

It has been noted that drug use is an attempt to mime, internally, the (to us external) structure, and effects, of our electronic environments—as it were, an attempt to play Perseus with the perceptions. Finnegans Wake *accomplishes this, not with chemicals or with pot, but with language: Joyce is as Perseus, the* Wake *his mirror (or "square wheel without spokes" which closes the time-gap of conscious-subconscious, of cognition and re-cognition) and ours for discerning, contending with and ultimately managing/ controlling/programming our psychic as well as social environments and responses.*
—ERIC MCLUHAN

Further Resources

See Eric McLuhan's *The Role of Thunder in Finnegans Wake*. See also A. Burgess's abridged version of the *Wake*, his study of Joyce, *Rejoyce*, and, of course, the complete *Finnegans Wake*. See the *Book of Highs* Spotify playlist for a recording of Joyce reading from the *Wake*. Other books that describe and analyze the happenings in the *Wake* include: *A Skeleton Key to Finnegans Wake* by Joseph Campbell and Henry Morton Robinson; *James Joyce: A Critical Introduction* by Harry Levin; and *A Reader's Guide to James Joyce* by William York Tindall.

185 Incense

An ancient technique to alter the nose.

Incense can be any aromatic substance that is burned in order to produce an odor. Incense is one of the best devices ever made for "altering" the nose. Be sure to smell the incense before you light it. Many different kinds of incense are available, and they all have a distinct odor both before and during consumption. Try many different kinds for different moods.

186 Sensory orgy

Feast on sights, smells, sounds, and textures.

Take as many different things as you can think of and lay them out in an open space where everyone can freely get at them. Invite some friends to take part in a feast for the perceptions. A sense orgy can be anything that will help you revel in your own sensory apparatus.

Spices work very well, as do different kinds of fabrics, synthetics, stones, water, incense, oils, foods, sand, earth, skins and pelts, sticks, bells, and so forth. Wearing a blindfold often heightens the sensations.

Further Resources

A very complete list of spices and their properties appears in Shirley "Wonderful" Ross's *The Interior Ecology Cookbook.*

187 Intensive instrument playing

Drum, blow, and play all day.

Music is a great consciousness alterer. If you can make music, do it all day and into the night. Drumming is especially useful in altering both breathing and blood circulation. Any wind instrument will definitely affect breathing in what can be a most extraordinary manner. String instruments, too, lend themselves well to changing consciousness, and cymbals are ideal. But nothing beats an organ.

· ·

188 Sound meditation
Sounds and vibrations can challenge and transport us.

For more than a decade, Alexandre Tannous has been exploring the possibility that sound can be an adjunct to meditation and also a source of altered states of consciousness. He has been researching the therapeutic and esoteric properties of sound from three different perspectives—Western scientific, Eastern philosophical, and shamanic societal beliefs—to gain a deeper understanding of how, and to what extent, sound has been used to affect human consciousness.

This search has led him to the intersection where art, science, and spirituality meet. His ethnomusicological approach entails a social scientific study of sound use in several traditional contexts—religious, spiritual, holistic, and cultural—for various purposes and occasions in entertainment, worship, meditation, and rituals of healing and trance. This has brought about a deeper understanding of how sound reveals and unlocks hidden powers we have within us to promote profound inner changes and healing.

Inspired by his findings, he designed a protocol of an integrated experience he calls "Sound Meditation" in which he shares the findings from his research, raising an awareness to how a specifically designed sound can have the ability to help us to disconnect from habitual patterns while judiciously listening to the specific traditional instruments he plays. He employs a phenomenological approach to study the effects of sound, using a method that empowers the participants to engage actively with tools that enhance their experience, using the consciousness-altering properties of sound to heighten self-awareness, to connect to the higher self, to fine-tune self-observation, and, perhaps, to attain self-realization.

The instruments he uses include gongs, bells, singing bowls, and a shruti box (a harmonium-like instrument that uses bellows and is often employed in Indian classical music to create a drone). Using the sounds produced by these instruments, he enables the listeners to disengage from habitual patterns by intentional listening.

Tannous says:

> Sound is mathematical and enigmatic. Sound can create sacred
> spaces inside of us. Tones, overtones and harmonics can lead
> us to sounds that fill the mind and can still the mind, leading to
> engagement and contemplation. These relationships between
> mathematics, harmonic series, and sounds relate to nature's
> harmonies: our breathing, our heart rate, and other physiological
> components. In my work, sounds are used in shamanic ways,
> analogous to the experiences with shamans where chants and
> drumming create spiritual resonances. When we lose ourselves in
> sound, the observer can disappear, and we can experience sounds
> that mold and tune the body and the mind through harmonies
> and sound symmetry.

The experience of sound meditation can be meditative, soothing, and, for
some, overwhelming. At a Tannous performance, I experienced the sounds
filling my consciousness. Though feeling somewhat overwhelmed by the
mixture of sounds and vibrations, I surrendered and followed them. I soon
felt transported to a serene type of consciousness alteration. Suddenly there
was a commotion in the room. Another woman in attendance was so overcome, she collapsed to the floor, no longer able to stand. As we rushed to
help her, we saw she was not only fully conscious and unharmed, but radi-
ating a shining and beatific smile.

Further Resources

See Tannous's website (soundmeditation.com).

• •

189 Metronome watching

A hypnotic trance.

A metronome is a device that marks time with a steady beat. The frequency of the beat is adjustable. There is usually a pendulum that swings
from side to side, marking the beat. The device is used in training for the
playing of musical instruments; it is also a most effective hypnotic induction device.

To begin watching a metronome, don't set it too fast or too slow; too fast and you won't be able to stay with it; too slow and you'll lose interest. But in the middle you should find your own beat. Watch it sway and swing, left, right, back, forth. Deeper, longer, heavier and heavier. You're getting sleepy. Your eyelids are so heavy you can hardly keep them up. You feel like closing your eyes and drifting off, off, off . . .

190 Stained glass

Contemplating beauty and divinity.

People go to church for a variety of reasons, many having to do with the alteration of consciousness. Yet our world has changed so much in the past century that it is difficult for churches to compete with all the other things in our environment: We just don't pay attention to church.

Seeing stained glass, however, is a profound experience. It was the ultimate expression of light for an entire epoch of history. To sit in a church for a day, watching the multifarious changes in color, hue, intensity; the subtlety with which the light plays—that was divinity. There is a different light show every day, and it runs on solar energy.

Further Resources

In Paris, go to Notre-Dame de Paris, and see especially the North Window. To sit in the cathedral at Chartres, France, reading Henry Adams's *Mont-St.-Michel and Chartres* as the light changes the windows, is a remarkable experience.

191 Hot and cold baths

Feel your body opening and closing.

Heat expands. Steam baths, sweat baths, saunas—they all open you up. As your pores open, whatever has been stopping them up flows out. This is cleansing, this is loosening. All heat allows you to move more.

Cold baths are deceptive. You probably think that the members of the local polar-bear club, the ones who get up at the crack of dawn in the winter to run and take a cold-water swim, are crazy. Could be; but they're also radically and swiftly changing their consciousness.

Cold baths are also great after a steam bath or a sauna. After you've finished sweating everything out, the cold water seals your skin tight. It feels great.

Further Resources

Sauna: The Finnish Bath tells you how to build it and use it properly. *Life in Harmony with Nature* by Adolf Hungry Wolf describes how to make an American Indian sweat bath.

192 Environmental control

Change a room's lighting, floor, and walls. How does it alter your experience?

Environmental control was pioneered by a group called USCO in the early 1960s. They recognized the fact that information is what shapes any environment. When you vary the information, say by adding more, creating an overload, then you change the environment. If you are aware of the changes they can be controlled.

Take a room and study the information that it dispenses. How does it feel? Sound? Smell? Taste? Look? If you change the covering on the floor you will change not just how the environment looks, but also how it sounds and how it feels. You will change the experience of the people who enter the new environment.

By changing images, lighting, and sound, and by keeping these changes in flow and in flux, you can control any environment so that there occurs consciousness alteration. Exterior decoration leads to interior alteration.

For major environmental control, build a dome, zome (a combination of a dome and zonohedron), or bubble over your space. It will really change everything.

Further Resources

Contact your local light-show group. For domes, check with Pacific Domes (pacificdomes.com).

. . . .

193 Sensory deprivation

Heightening awareness by limiting.

S ensory deprivation is the removal of as many sensory inputs as possible. Usually this is accomplished by the use of complicated equipment that blocks all light sources, soundproofs the environment, limits tactile sensation, and deprives the perceptual processes of any odors or tastes.

A variety of equipment has been used to accomplish sensory deprivation. The most common: a soundproof, lightproof chamber enclosing a bathtub-like tank. The subject of sensory "dep" enters the water-filled tank, which limits movement and creates a feeling of weightlessness (via Epsom salts) to greatly reduce tactile input, one of our most constant sources of sensory data. (We are generally not aware of this, living, as we do, in a highly visual culture. But as you read this you are probably touching the book, your clothing, some furniture, the ground, etc. This perceptual information tends to become background in our sensorily overloaded environment.) This kind of sensory dep can be tolerated for only short periods of time.

You can accomplish a limited amount of sensory dep yourself by finding a darkened closet, filling it with pillows, and making some ear baffles, a blindfold, and whatever else you feel will limit your sensory input. Make sure you will not be disturbed (unless you need help, which *must* always be present and available). Enter the closet and do your best to limit all movements, even twitching and scratching. Don't stay in for too long! Usually a couple of hours will produce effects that are both inescapable and dominant.

When you remove visual input you can expect, after a while, to experience new visual sensations, either hallucinations or, possibly, the appearance of phosphene patterns. When you limit auditory input, you can expect to hear sounds that are always there, but are overwhelmed by the sounds of the environment. You will hear your breathing, your heart, the circulation of blood in and around your ears, and a variety of other sounds. This seems quite simple, but never having really listened to these sounds before, you can experience them as deafening and overpowering. They never stop.

When sensory data from the environment is cut out and inner sensory data becomes available, it can often be frightening. Many people who have taken part in sensory dep experiments have had unpleasant experiences. There is evidence, however, that the manner in which the researcher presents and administers the experiment greatly shape and determine the subject's experience.

Still, to distance the experience from the negative associations of the past, sensory deprivation tanks are now often called "floatation tanks" or "Restricted Environmental Stimulation Therapy" (REST).

Many people who participated in long-term experiments (lasting more than twenty-four hours) found relief from the negative effects of SD by sleeping and playing games and engaging in mental exercises (learning the alphabet backward, solving mathematical problems, etc.). Once sleep time was exhausted and the exercises could no longer be maintained, the subjects would demand to be released. Most people find SD intolerable. Without proper controls it can be dangerous. Proceed carefully.

Further Resources

Sensory deprivation tanks have experienced a resurgence recently, with several centers appearing in New York, Portland, San Francisco, and other cities. Check your local listings to find one near you. The original standard text on the subject is *Sensory Deprivation* by Solomon, Kubzansky, Leiderman, Mendelson, and Wexler. John C. Lilly, inventor of the sensory deprivation tank, also wrote a book on his findings and experiences: *The Deep Self: Consciousness Exploration in the Isolation Tank.*

194 Witches' cradle and ASCID

A torture device from the Inquisition becomes a tool for altering consciousness.

According to the historical accounts of some witches, Inquisitors would place the accused inside a bag that would be strung up over a limb of a tree. This made the bag swing in a pendulum-like motion while the witch inside was confined and in a sensory-deprivation-like position. The witches then adapted this procedure, known as the Witches' Cradle, for their "transportation" to the "Witches' Sabbat."

The first attempt to rebuild the Witches' Cradle for achieving altered states was made by Robert Masters and Jean Houston. Their Altered State of Consciousness Induction Device (ASCID) is a metal swing in which the subject stands upright. This swinglike container tends to sway to and fro, and left and right, greatly exaggerating the movement of the occupant. The occupant is strapped into the ASCID and is blindfolded. Some experimenters also use ear baffles. Most people who try an ASCID experience an altered

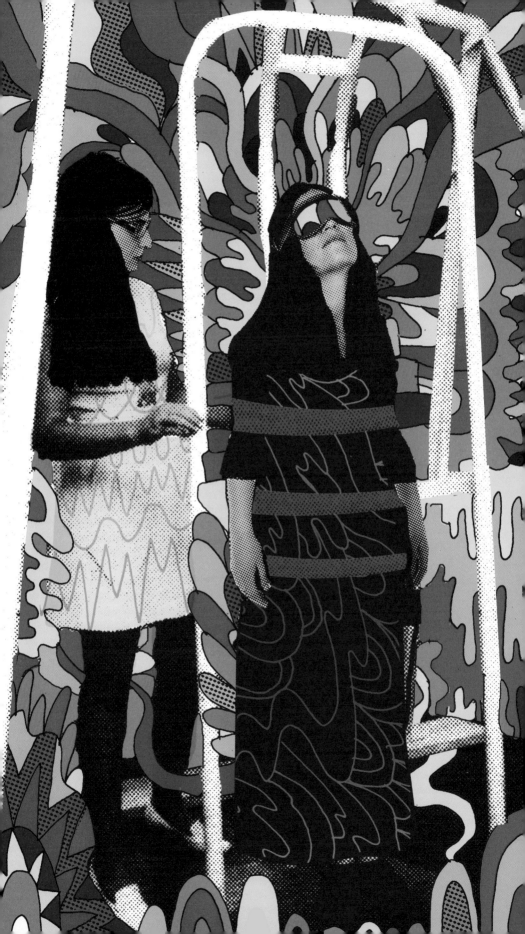

state of consciousness, characterized by increased visual imagery and by highly realistic fantasy trips to other places, other lands, and other worlds. The altered state usually begins within twenty minutes.

Recently, art collectives have been building renditions of the Witches' Cradle that are closer to those described in the witches' accounts. The Toronto-based Center for Tactical Magic offered an interactive exhibit with the devices in 2009. As their website states: "Cradles create a place where one can begin to realize an altered state (of consciousness, or an altered political state) and contemplate the next course of action."

Further Resources

The work of Masters and Houston with the Witches' Cradle is described in their *New Ways of Being*. Some mention of the experiments is in their book mentioned in the resources for No. 148. Bernard Aaronson and others at the New Jersey Neuropsychiatric Institute also conducted a study with their horizontal ASCID. The Center for Tactical Magic features videos of their Witches' Cradles in action on their website (tacticalmagic.org).

. . . .

195 Body confinement

Limiting movement can create new sensations.

Most body confinement takes place as a result of medical procedures. It used to be confinement in a respirator due to polio or respiratory ailments, and is currently experienced in confinement in traction or in body casts. All of these devices create a sensory deprivation experience, because of the reduction of sensory input. Auditory and visual hallucinations are often reported.

Other kinds of body confinement are described in what is known as the bondage branch of erotic literature. Many people derive sexual pleasure from being tied and bound so that they are totally confined and unable to move. Havelock Ellis wrote that the restraint of emotional and physical activity tends to heighten sexual excitement. There are many kinds of confinement that are used in bondage and discipline pursuits including totally encircling a person's entire body in sturdy wrapping tape, the kind used for packaging.

196–199
VISUAL ILLUSIONS

What you see as "reality" isn't always real.

Color. Movement. Angle. Shape. Dimensions. Our brains process an incredible amount of visual data every second. Sometimes, when this data is limited, our brains fill in gaps. Prisoner's cinema is a fine example—when total darkness eliminates visual input, your brain will generate wild light shows of its own making. Sometimes, when there is too much or conflicting input, our brains will struggle and also generate images that are not truly "there." While humans have some of the finest eyesight in the animal kingdom, our perception of the world is still an approximation—and subject to error. Here are a few illusions that reveal both the power and the limits of our brains. Remember: What you see as "reality" isn't always real.

Further Resources

All of the illusions below can be found online. Books filled with optical tricks and explanations abound—see especially *Eye and Brain: The Psychology of Seeing* by Richard Gregory and *Masters of Deception: Escher, Dalí & the Artists of Optical Illusion* by Al Seckel. For examples of autostereograms (No. 198), one need only consult the myriad Magic Eye books available.

••

196 Hermann's grid

At every intersection of the white lines, our eyes perceive a gray dot. When you look directly at one of the intersections though, the dot disappears.

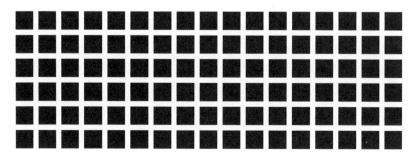

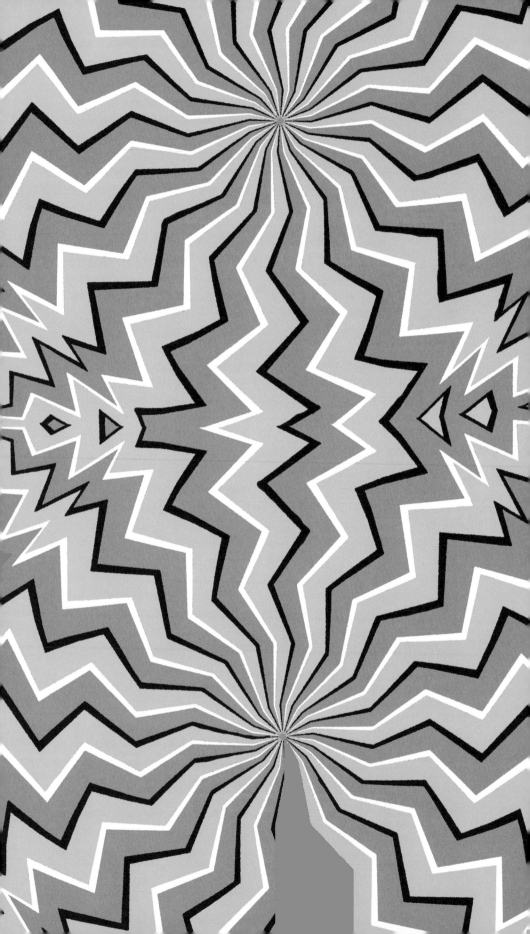

197 Peripheral drift

V ery popular in the op art movement, kinetic illusions are stationary images that give the appearance of motion. Peripheral drift is a fine example of this phenomenon. As a result of the angles and interplay of black and white, your eyes lose their place and in refocusing make the image appear to move. Look slightly to the side of this image on the left. The swirls should appear to turn.

198 Autostereo-grams

A utostereograms play tricks on your depth perception. They present repeating two-dimensional patterns with an embedded image. In order to focus on both the embedded image and the repeating patterns, our brain will situate them on two different planes—with the embedded image either floating above or below the pattern, in 3D. The popular Magic Eye illusions are examples of autostereograms.

199 Ames perceptual demonstrations

Objects, even people, are bigger—or smaller!—than they appear.

E ven when we know that what we are perceiving is not true, we still perceive it. This sounds like a riddle, but actually it was what led Adelbert Ames Jr. to construct a number of perceptual-demonstration devices so that we could see just how our senses often perceive that which is not actually present in the environment. For example, Ames designed a distorted room, which appears cubic—though it is actually a trapezoid—and flat—though it is actually on an incline with walls that slant outward. When two people stand on opposite sides and a third looks into the room via a peephole, it appears that one is enormously larger than the other. Even when we know the truth about what the demonstration shows, it is impossible to inhibit the experience of the illusory or distorted image.

200 Mandalas

The universe in miniature.

M andalas are circular images often used as devices to alter consciousness and to increase awareness, especially during meditation. The Tibetan Buddhists used their religious paintings of mandalas, known as tankas or thangkas, as models for the universe in miniature. Other cultures have used the mandala form in art, architecture, and dance as means of expressing wholeness. The earth and the moon and the sun are mandalas. The clearest images that we have of atoms and their constituent entities are in the mandala form, as are galaxies and galactic systems like the Milky Way.

Most mandalas used for meditation have centers so that the meditator has a point on which to focus, to concentrate their efforts and energies. Then by letting their own energy move out from the center of the mandala they can experience the movement of energy, through form-taking, throughout the cosmos.

Further Resources

R obert E. L. Masters and Jean Houston's *Psychedelic Art* contains some interesting mandalas and some examples of the works of artists of the "fantastic realism" school whose paintings may assist in changing consciousness. Giuseppe Tucci's *The Theory and Practice of the Mandala* is most complete. Jung's *The Archetypes and the Collective Unconscious* contains mandalas drawn by patients who were using the form as a means of self-expression and self-discovery. Some of the paintings were done by Jung himself. José and Miriam Argüelles have produced a beautiful book devoted to the subject of circular paintings and images called *Mandala*.

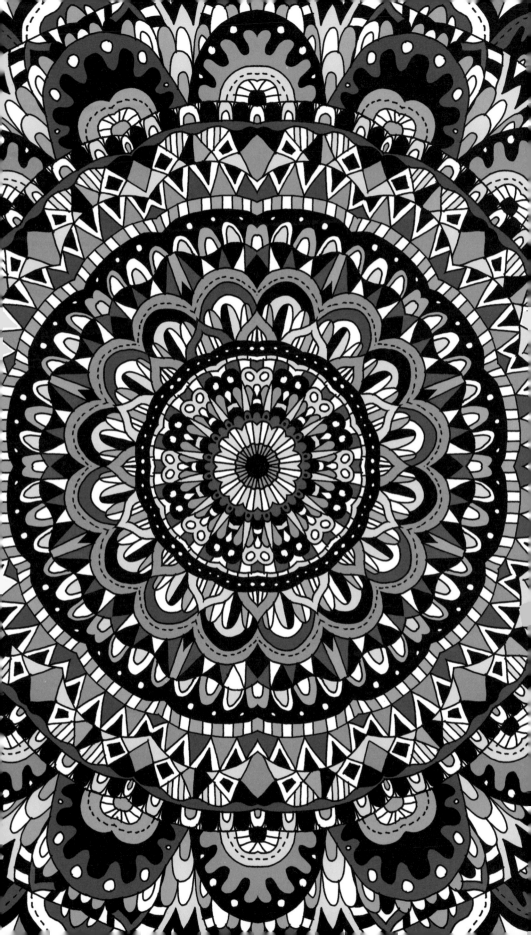

· ·

201 Gymnastic equipment
A playground for all ages.

It's hard to get higher than you get on a trampoline.

Bouncing around in the sky.

Jumping and floating and almost flying.

Rings. Swings.

Seesaws and trapezes.

They're all great.

Ask any kid.

· ·

202 Scuba and skin diving
The sensory delights of the deep.

Skin diving takes you down into another world, right here on earth. People who go to the moon are called astronauts of outer space; many who delve into their own minds are called astronauts of inner space. Perhaps skin divers and others who go deep into the sea should be called astronauts of under space.

The planet Earth is 80 percent water. Species unfamiliar to your eye exist by the thousands in the oceans and seas of the world. Using the proper gear and technique, a technique that can be learned in schools throughout the United States, you can explore this world with all of its sensory delights and mind-boggling sights and experiences.

Technically, skin diving is underwater swimming with a snorkel breathing device; SCUBA stands for Self-Contained Underwater Breathing Apparatus.

203 Bells

Ringing a real bell is a full-body experience.

Ringing bells can get you high. The bigger the bell, the better. In the old world the ringing of bells was the focal point and ordering process of town life. But those were real bells, with tone and intensity, not like our school bells and alarm clocks, which sound dull, thudding, and mechanical.

Get yourself some real bells; current technology-produced bell sounds are no substitute. Large ones are best, but small ones are good, too. Ring them and listen for the special sound that will make you feel the bell's vibrations and your own.

204 Masks

What do you become when you wear the face of another?

The wearing of masks is a definite device for the alteration of consciousness. This is true both for the wearer of the mask and for the one who perceives the masked figure. Think of the Lone Ranger, of the Noh theater of Japan, of Halloween, and you may gather the strength of mask wearing. The mask is often symbolic of desired powers or attributes, often worn in tribes to show members the power the wearer has gained by donning the mask of an animal or spirit.

Pick a spirit, mythological character, animal, or creature with whom you identify; or ask your friends to pick one that they think fits you. Then go and make up a mask that you feel conveys the feelings of that character. Make it out of paper, clay, tinfoil, or papier-mâché, or simply paint your face with water-based paints.

When you can be alone, wear the mask. See the power that it gives you. Feel the energy of the creature portrayed by its image enter you.

Further Resources

See Jung's *Man and His Symbols* for an interesting discussion of the use of masks and the mask as persona.

· ·

205 Rock throwing

A simple, satisfying outlet for anger.

R ock throwing can be one of the most fulfilling ways to express your anger. You can throw rocks against other rocks (watch out for the fly-ing particles). You can throw rocks against the ground. You can throw rocks into the water, much like the shot put in athletic competition. You can rip weeds out of the ground or express your fury by shredding up dead leaves.

In some Malaysian tribes, people express their anger in a most ecologi-cally unsound manner: They hack at trees. When a tribesman becomes angry, he goes out into the jungle and hacks at the trees until a trance-frenzy devel-ops, allowing for complete catharsis. Then he can return to the tribe with a more balanced life attitude.

· ·

206 Automobile destruction

Where exertion and a forbidden activity create a thrilling state.

E cologically sound, and possibly even cathartic after a day spent in bumper-to-bumper traffic. Required: open space, an automobile, implements of destruction (e.g., sledgehammer, ax, club, crowbar, acetylene torch, etc.). Be careful: Automobiles may be dangerous to your health; this is true for their destruction also. (There is danger of being injured by flying pieces of bro-ken glass or being cut by shredded metal.) This may be the Western answer to hacking at trees. Destroy a car. Make sure that you recycle all the junk.

This kind of behavior induces an altered state of consciousness as a result of the sheer effort, the intense breathing that takes place, and the psy-chological experience of both destruction and the forbidden.

207 Kayak disease

Long periods on the water create horrible hallucinations.

Next time you're in Greenland, if you go out hunting in a kayak and you stay out for more than three days, well, that's usually when kayak disease sets in. Terrible hallucinations, both auditory and visual, may affect you; extreme disorientation may also ensue. Be careful.

Further Resources

Also known as "kayak angst" and "kayak-dizziness," kayak disease is described in Daniel Merkur's *Becoming Half Hidden: Shamanism and Initiation Among the Inuit*, as well as *Scientific American*'s 2009 article "Foreign Afflictions: Mental Disorders across Country Borders." Although out of print, L. LeCron's *Experimental Hypnosis* features a nice article, "Hypnosis in Perspective," by G. W. Williams that addresses the phenomenon.

208 Engine rough

On especially long drives, the sound of your engine may be dangerously hypnotic.

Engine rough is part of the highway- or road-hypnosis experience. It is usually encountered by truck drivers or others who must spend long hours on the road. Engine rough is the auditory sensation that occurs from overexposure to a repetitive engine sound. Its effects are very similar to those of other auditory hallucinations. Highway hypnosis is worse than falling asleep at the wheel. The trance produced is usually not corrected merely by awakening. It is especially prevalent and dangerous when driving during rain, hail, sleet, or snow.

What happens is that the constant, repetitious sound of the engine forms background noise, much like music. Out of this background come other sounds, all of which are illusions. These sounds range from human voices to automobile-horn blowing. The effects can be very dangerous. Similar sensations occur to the fatigued driver, though he might just fall asleep. Engine rough can cause a driver to react to the illusory sensations, often provoking accidents and shock reaction. It is not recommended that you pursue this altered state of consciousness.

· ·

209 Skydiving

You are flying!

As if in a dream, the clouds surround you, birds fly by, you see the roads and rooftops and people below. The wind envelopes you in what feels like a protective shield as you hurtle earthward. You're picking up speed and the ground below seems to be flying, heading up toward you with great speed. You are truly flying. Then, suddenly, a jolt and everything is pulling you upward, if only for a few seconds. Now, your speed is slowing. Is it a dream? No. Your parachute has opened—thank God!—and you have been safely skydiving.

For eons, humans have wanted to fly like birds, to leave the ground and soar through the air. Ballooning was the first instance where this became possible, and the development of parachutes soon followed.

Leonardo da Vinci sketched an image of a parachute in one of his notebooks and the idea sparked people to think about flying safely through the air. The first practical parachute was invented by Louis-Sébastien Lenormand. He put together two umbrellas and jumped out of a tree in 1783. The first parachute jump, from a balloon at a height of more than 3,000 feet, came in 1797, performed by André-Jacques Garnerin, who studied the concept of resistance of the air to slow objects and people falling from high altitudes.

Then, in the last century, planes appeared and enabled humans to fly, if not quite the way birds do. Combining working planes that flew safely and the parachute brought about the ability to dive through the sky and then parachute down to the Earth's solid ground, without injury or death: skydiving. The first ripcord-operated parachute jump was performed by Leslie Irvin in 1919. Since then, the many methods of skydiving have made it an international sport. Skydiving facilities exist in many area airports.

There are risks, of both injuries and even death. This is not a sport for the fainthearted, though one-hundred-year-old skydivers often make the news with videos of their exploits. The latest incarnation of skydiving is groups who skydive in increasingly complex formations.

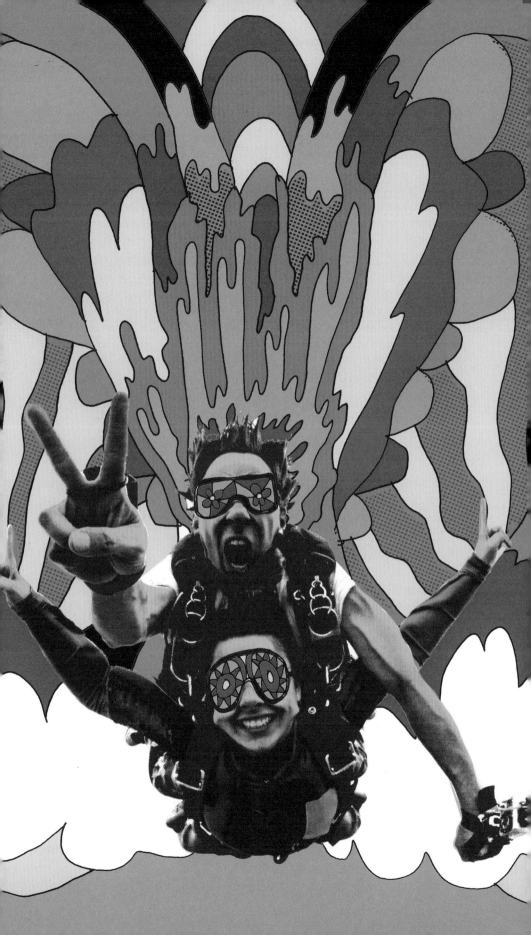

210 Breakoff

Hallucinations experienced by high-altitude pilots.

A breakoff phenomenon is peculiar to high-altitude jet pilots. It is a form of sensory deprivation, with the usual accompanying hallucinatory experiences, and is a result of lack of orientation points and stimuli at high altitudes.

When flying through weather of high barometric pressure, that is, empty, cloudless skies, or when flying for extended periods on instruments through intense cloud cover, the pilot has, literally, nothing to look at except the inside of the cockpit. Often the hallucinations involve movement illusions, since breakoff takes place when the pilot cannot tell whether or not he is moving.

Further Resources

A. M. H. Bennett has written the authoritative article "Sensory Deprivation in Aviation," which appeared in *Sensory Deprivation* by Solomon et al.

211 Gliding

A near-silent journey through the sky.

G liding is different from flying because of the almost total silence it involves. The only sound heard, as you soar on the wind currents and air pockets, is the air itself as it whooshes over the wings and past the cabin. Also known as sailplaning and soaring, gliding allows for incredible experiences: altitudes of more than 45,000 feet, speeds of more than 160 miles per hour, and some of the most fantastic dives in all aviation. You can glide for more than 600 miles without landing.

The way to soar is to locate a soaring club and complete training, including any examinations required. You can then buy, rent, or borrow a glider and hitch up behind a small engine-powered plane that will tow you up to at least 3,000 feet and then let you go. Then just steer your way toward a thermal current so you can join the birds.

212 Land diving

A thrilling rite of passage.

O n Pentecost Island in the South Pacific, when a man has something he wants to get off his chest, when he has something that he wants to tell all of his fellow tribesmen, he climbs to the top of an eighty-three-foot tower, affixes spring vines around his ankles, and holds one hand above his head. This is the signal that he wishes to speak, and the dancing and singing some eight stories below him come to a halt. All are attentive to the complaint or cry or story. It might be that he has paid too high a price for a pig or is very proud to be a member of the tribe.

After finishing his speech, he raises both hands above his head, claps them three times, and dives head first toward the softened earth some eighty feet below him. As his head reaches the soft earth, specially prepared for his landing place, the vines (called lianas) attached to his ankles snap tight, and the platform above collapses from the strain to absorb the shock of the fall. His head barely touches the earth as he rebounds and is held tight by the vines, swinging in an arc.

This surely must be one of the most extraordinary ways of altering consciousness.

Further Resources

K al Muller tried land diving in the New Hebrides, on Pentecost Island, and told about it in the December 1970 *National Geographic*. *National Geographic* also made a television special on these islands that included a sequence on land diving. It is available on *The Book of Highs* YouTube playlist.

213 Skiing and snowboarding

Sliding through the snow.

S kiing and snowboarding, with their speed and grace, are fine ways to alter consciousness and sharpen perceptual awareness. What contributes to all of this is the heightened experience brought on by the extreme cold, the dazzling brightness of the sun, and the sensorily deprived experience one has in being in such a pure white environment.

As you whoosh through the snow, your skis or board will make a smooth churning sound as they carry you speedily on your way; you feel your body smoothly steering you as it twists, turns, bends, and stretches. You become your skis, your board, the snow.

• •

214 Space travel

The final frontier.

> In an airplane, during the day, the sky is, of course, still blue, no matter how high you go. If you fly higher you see further, so that is not unexpected. But the first thing that hit me with this view was that it was daylight, we were flying over the sunlit side of the Earth, yet most of what we saw out the window was the pitch blackness of empty space. It didn't matter that I've seen it this way on *Star Trek* or any other science fiction movie a thousand times. Seeing so much blackness, while seeing the Earth so brightly lit, was a contrast that surprised me more than expected. Although we are not so far away from the Earth in this orbit, different from being in an aircraft, the sensation was of two objects, our ship and the Earth, both floating in a dark void. And then there was another feeling. It wasn't that the Earth looked small, in fact it looks huge—the biggest thing you've ever seen—but from here you can see its shape, its size, and you get a gut feeling of being able to measure it with your own eyes. It's not the view, but this feeling that goes with it, of being able to measure it, that really washed over me.
> —GREG CHAMITOFF, US ASTRONAUT AND FLIGHT ENGINEER

This is what is called the "overview effect" that many astronauts and cosmonauts report upon seeing the planet Earth from space. It is a mind altering state, with weightlessness and other aspects of space travel adding to the feelings they experience of otherworldliness. Upon seeing, live, the tiny blue sphere, the blue marble, or the enormous Earth, these space travelers see our planet in its true light, "hanging in the void," with nourishment only from a super-thin, almost paper-like layer of atmosphere shielding

Earth from space. Ian O'Neill's "The Human Brain in Space: Euphoria and the 'Overview Effect' Experienced in Astronauts" put it best: "From space, national boundaries vanish, the conflicts that divide people become less important, and the need to create a planetary society with the united will to protect this 'pale blue dot' becomes both obvious and imperative."

Further Resources

A simple web search will bring up the accounts of many astronauts describing what it was like for them when they traveled in space. Entrepreneurs including Jeff Bezos, Richard Branson, and Elon Musk have all announced plans for letting civilians go into space, with the promise of returning to Earth.

215 Trepanning
Does drilling a hole in your head get you high?

Trepanation is an ancient process, an operation whereby a hole is drilled in the head and part of the skull is removed. This is done in order to increase the volume of blood that reaches the brain. Bart Hughes of Amsterdam claimed that the operation would not only make anyone undergoing it "high" for life, but would also cure all mental illness.

Further Resources

T. Lobsang Rampa describes his pre- and post-trepanation experiences in *The Third Eye*. Bart Hughes wrote of his experience in his autobiography, *The Book with the Hole*.

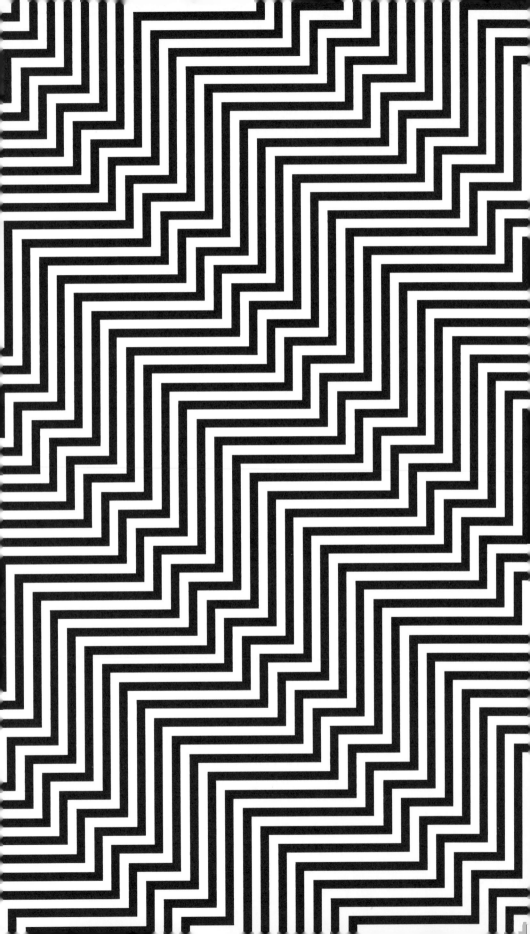

CHAPTER 9

ELECTRIC

The only difference between a drug and a computer is that one is slightly too large to swallow. . . . And our best people are working on that problem, even as we speak.

—TERENCE MCKENNA

. . . .

216 Sensory overload

Faced with information overload, we have no alternative but pattern recognition.
—MARSHAL McLUHAN

Just as our sensory equipment reacts when we deny it data from the environment, it will create an entirely different reaction when overloaded with environmental data. In speaking of Sensory Deprivation in No. 193, I mentioned that the senses cue in on internal information when cut off from the usual flow of sensation produced by the environment. Internal sensations are usually distinguished and experienced as hallucination, illusion, distortion of "normal" perception, and disorientation. With sensory overload, some of these same sensations appear, only in different forms and configurations.

Our cognitive apparatus is constantly selecting and screening the stimuli that bombard us from the environment. We focus our attention on one figure, image, or event, and the other perceptions fall into a background configuration. Sensory overload is the state that occurs when so many images and sounds are competing to become the center of our attention that we are unable, consciously or unconsciously, to make a choice. We are overwhelmed, carried off by the stream and flow of bombarding imagery and sensation. We literally don't know where to turn.

This state can lead to visual and auditory hallucinations (seeing and hearing things that do not originate from given stimuli), illusion (taking given stimuli from the environment and perceptually misapprehending them so as to change their nature), and extreme disorientation. Occasionally, sensory overload leads to creative breakthroughs, increased mental imagery, problem solving, synesthesias (see No. 83), and even to psychotic experiences.

The major social examples of sensory overload are the light shows that accompany concerts. Some planetariums and movie theaters have incorporated concepts of sensory overload into their productions. The fully immersive IMAX and 3-D experiences are two modern examples. Many people consider some aspects of contemporary global urban life—increased activity, lights from advertising displays, and overwhelming noise pollution—to create a permanent state of overload, even for those who do not desire to exist under such conditions.

Decades ago, a good example of the deliberately constructed sensory overload environment was at the Foundation for Mind Research then located in New York City, but since closed. Robert Masters and Jean Houston, with the help of lumia artist Don Snyder, created a total audiovisual environment, as well as a portable audiovisual-olfactory-tactile device.

The environment was composed of an 8 x 8–foot semicircular rear–projection screen. The subject sat behind the screen, very close to the center of its curve. In this way, the visual images would occupy her/his total field of vision and the sensation of being "in" the images was accomplished. The visual images were from 2 x 2–inch or 35mm slides. The slide-projecting equipment was computer-controlled and linked to the sound track either through a set of individual headphones or through speakers situated on either side. The rate of speed of the dissolve, that is, the intervals at which the slides changed and new images were shown on the screen, varied from one to twenty seconds. The slide changes were geared to the sound track.

For software in the visual area, the foundation used slides hand painted in transparent colors, so that many slides were original works of art. Images from such painters as Bosch, Breughel, Fuchs, Klarwein, and Tchelitchew were also shown. The sound track was usually electronic music augmented by Zen and Sufi chanting.

The foundation had also developed an environmental overload device that made it possible to control and overload visual, auditory, olfactory, and tactile stimulation. This device was like a small version of the curved rear screen, except that it was shaped like an elongated bubble that fits over the head. When images were projected on the head covering, the subject was, literally, inside of the pictures being presented: The images formed a total surround. There were earphones inside of the device as well as a series of air hoses. These hoses not only brought fresh air to the subject but could also be used both to introduce odors and to change the flow of air speed, thereby altering the tactile experience.

This device remained in the experimental stage. It was imagined, that, when completed, all of the different sensations would be computer-controlled so that when the Tibetan tanka mandala image filled the visual field, the chanting would get louder over the sound track, the odor of temple incense would fill the device, and the air would come rushing at the subject's face timed to the beats of the chant.

Virtual reality headgear currently can be programmed to approximate similar kinds of sensory overload experiences (see No. 246).

Further Resources

William Sargant's *Battle for the Mind* and Perry London's *Behavior Control* discuss the more formal aspects of sensory overload and bombardment. Other Masters and Houston references may be found in Nos. 148 and 194.

· ·

217 Electronic dance music

A modern world trance ritual.

The tremendous space, usually an empty warehouse or similar large building, is filled with people, as many as a thousand or thousands. They're all moving together, dancing, jumping up and down. The music is possessed by that insistent beat: *thump, thump, thump, thump. . . .* You can feel the beat inside your body and inside everyone's bodies around you as you move and gyrate. The melody and rhythm build and build, until breaking in an orgasmic release. And the lights, the patterns, the colors, moving and changing so constantly, an intergalactic light show playing out all around you . . . it's really a sensory overload experience.

Electronic dance music (EDM) helps to create altered states of consciousness, of awareness, of yourself and others, and of your body and all the other dancers' bodies, all seemingly in a trance. Their success—in 2014 more than half of concert ticket sales worldwide were for EDM shows—speaks to the power of these experiences.

Listening to EDM can be enjoyable, but to truly get high from the experience, you probably have to attend a live show.

Further Resources

Check your local concert listing for an EDM performance near you.

· ·

218 Natural sound amplification

Use a stethoscope and microphone to "broadcast" your internal music.

You are constantly making noise. Your heart beats and pumps as your lungs fill and collapse. The blood rushes through your veins and arteries. You breathe. If you've ever had your head in anyone's lap for a sufficient amount of time, you know that the stomach and intestines do not go about their procedures in total silence. Your bones screech and creak, and occasionally crack. When you scratch your skin, your nails make cacophonic symphonies.

The stethoscope is the best instrument available for listening to sounds within the body. All of the noises noted above can be made clearly audible with a stethoscope. But what is really an extraordinary experience is to connect a stethoscope to a sensitive microphone and amplification equipment and "broadcast" your own internal music.

John Cage describes entering an echoic chamber, a totally soundproofed room. He heard two sounds, one high, the other low. When he discussed these sounds with the engineer in charge, Cage was told that the high sound was that of his nervous system and the low one that of his blood circulating.

Further Resources

A stethoscope may be purchased at any medical supply center. As suggested in No. 154, sounds coming through a speaker may be used as a massage. Amplification of natural body sounds will serve this purpose as well as chanting. John Cage's story comes from his lecture "Experimental Music" in his book *Silence*.

219 Prolonged radar-screen observation

When time and limited sensory input cause illusions.

Watching a radar screen is a form of sensory deprivation. What is most alarming about radar-screen watching is that after several hours even the most competent operators see blips that aren't there.

220 Movies

From IMAX to 3D to YouTube, movies are more and more actively designed to make you turn on.

There you are, sitting in near-total darkness, surrounded by a large crowd that has gathered to participate in a highly ritualized social event. The main content of this event is to watch larger-than-life images as they are projected on a screen and reflected back to your eyes. All of this is done in relative silence.

The future of cinema is, in many ways, already here. IMAX and other successful 3D experiences enable the viewer to feel fully centered and enveloped by the cinematic display. This heightens feelings of transformation, being "there," being swept away, much further and faster, into the movie's content and imagery. With animation, this can lead to an expanded sense of belief, where cartoonlike imagery seems to be quite real, virtually alive. Advances in audio processing and speaker placements, as well as light-field changes in cinematic projection are on the horizon. The future of how we see, hear, and experience movies seems without limits.

But this isn't the first time filmmakers have tapped into the medium's power to alter consciousness. From stroboscopes to spiritual journeys, from zooming into our bodies to zooming out into the cosmos, movies utilize sight, sound, and motion to reveal what's inside ourselves and beyond. Here are a few examples of my favorite consciousness-altering films.

Flicker Film by Tony Conrad is a good example. This is a short subject that uses frames of pure white and black, alternating on the screen, to produce a stroboscopic flicker effect. Most people watching the first few minutes of the film are bored and start to complain. But after about five minutes the white and black images flickering on the screen make the viewer begin to see colors where there are none. What Conrad has done is to create a film that stimulates the eye, the optic nerve, and the brain to produce its own color.

Other interesting films include those made by the Whitney brothers, who produced short subjects of computer-generated mandala patterns that changed and transformed with great intricate motions. Alejandro Jodorowsky's *El Topo* portrays a man's search for a master within himself by his meetings with masters of the Yogic, Gurdjieffian, Sufistic, and Taoistic persuasions. Peter Brook's screen version of *Marat/Sade* brings madness to life on the screen. Chris Munger's short *X-Ray Film* takes you on a journey inside your own body. Charles Eames's *Powers of Ten* takes you from a picnic table in Florida out to the farthest reaches of the cosmos in the space of less than 10 minutes.

Further Resources

Gene Youngblood's *Expanded Cinema* gives further details on the link between cinema and consciousness. Here are some films that will change almost everyone's consciousness—all are available on the *Book of Highs* YouTube playlist, except where otherwise noted. *The Powers of Ten* (Charles Eames's adaptation of Boeke's book *Cosmic View,* eight minutes that transport you visually to the outer ranges of the universe); *Flicker Film* (Tony and Beverly Conrad's film, shot entirely in black and white, makes most viewers see colors, much like stroboscopic phenomena); *Binary Bit Patterns* (by Michael Whitney and available at archive.org); *Crystals* (Herbert Loebel's film of microphotography); and *X-Ray Film* (Chris Munger's view of how man functions, from inside; available on vimeo.com).

• •

221 Stroboscopes

From your home to the lab to the dance floor, a classic hallucinatory experience.

Stroboscopes are devices that create pulsations of light at regular and fixed intervals varying from one flash for every several seconds to several flashes per second. In order to experience hallucinations, one sits in front of a stroboscope with the eyes closed. When the machine is turned on, the flashes of light should be aimed at the closed eyes. The stroboscope's varying speed mechanism should be set between 8 and 25 flashes per second. It is in this area that most people experience visual images. The speed that generates the most images is 10 flashes per second. The varying of speed will vary the images produced.

The above instructions apply only to the xenon strobe. This strobe produces a type of "artificial lightning," a very bright flash of white-to-violet light. Another, older type of strobe produces a different form of sensation. This is the neon strobe, which produces a reddish light that is not as bright as the light flashes of the xenon strobe. With the red-lighted neon strobe, hallucinatory effects are possible with the eyes *open*.

When the strobe is flashing at the speeds indicated above, the observer will notice an image that seems to float just above the strobe. This image will vary in color through the entire red-to-green section of the spectrum as the speed of stroboscopic flash is varied.

Stroboscopes are used in the laboratory to divide motion activity into discrete elements, making the object illuminated appear not to be in motion. The same effect will be gained if you or anyone you please is placed under strobe illumination. You will appear not to be moving when you are. All of your motions will be broken down and frozen in time. Dance clubs use strobes to illuminate the dance floor for just this purpose.

Further Resources

Strobes are sold wherever equipment for light shows is sold, at theatrical equipment houses, and through scientific-instrument supply centers. Finding an old neon strobe just takes hunting around. Or you can put a red shield over the face of a xenon strobe, which will make it approximate the effects of a neon model. A strobe that synchronizes its flashing with your brain waves is called the Brain Wave Synchronizer.

• •

222 Continuous light and sound

What happens when you live in a world of sound and light 24/7?

Continuous light and sound environments were the work of La Monte Young and Marian Zazeela. In decades past, they maintained, at their studio in New York City, an environment of constant-periodic sound-wave forms generated by an electronic synthesizer. Young had analyzed a series of rational-frequency ratios and would adjust his synthesizer so that a number of frequencies were sounded constantly. These frequencies, somewhat like electronic chords to the ear, were played at the Young-Zazeela studio-home twenty-four hours a day, seven days a week, starting in September 1966 and continuing at least until the 1970s. They worked, played, ate, talked, socialized, slept, dreamed, and made love while these frequencies filled the air. Young and Zazeela call this kind of sound environment "House Hums."

In addition to these constant, ever-present frequencies, the studio was always in a state of flux with a variety of moving and alternating lighting effects. Some lights would go on and off, others changed color, tone, intensity, and hue (as did the sounds, when Young adjusted the synthesizer). It took about twenty minutes to get "high" in the studio, just from the flux of light-and-sound frequencies. When desired, alteration of consciousness could be achieved in seconds, by specific changes in frequency.

Other continuous light and sound environments have been designed and executed by Robert Masters, Jean Houston, and Don Snyder.

Further Resources

A search for La Monte Young and Marian Zazeela on the Web will bring up a variety of written, audio, and video resources related to their pioneering works. Their *Selected Writings* is still available. Masters and Houston used to maintain their environment at their Institute for Mind Research in New York, now closed.

· ·

223 Dream machine

Build your own flicker instrument.

Inspired by W. Gray Walter's book *The Living Brain*, which detailed the effects of stroboscopic flicker phenomena in producing hallucinations, Ian Sommerville and Brion Gysin devised the Dream Machine.

The Dream Machine is a homemade flicker-producing instrument. All that is necessary to make it is some cardboard or poster paper, a light bulb, and a turntable that will revolve at 78 rpm.

Make a cylinder 10 inches high from the cardboard. Make sure that the cylinder will fit on the turntable. Then cut ten horizontal slots, five each on opposite sides of the cylinder. The slots should each be 1½ inches apart and measure about 4 inches long and ⅜ of an inch wide.

Suspend an electric light bulb (100 watts incandescent; 26 watts CFL) inside the cylinder on the turntable. Be sure the light bulb is level with the slots in the cylinder. Start the turntable at 78 rpm so that the cylinder

revolves at this speed. The bulb is stationary. Bring your *closed* eyes as close to the slots as possible. You will see images similar to those produced by a xenon strobe.

Further Resources

Kristian Nielsen wrote about his experience making a Dream Machine, along with instructions, in *Vice* magazine in 2016 ("I Tried to Trip on Light with My Homemade Dream Machine").

· ·

224 Riley room

A hall of echoes.

Terry Riley, a musician and environmental artist who has worked with La Monte Young, constructed a most ingenious room of images and repetition. Within the walls of the room are about nine different outer chambers and one central chamber. All of the chambers are connected by doors that lead to the other chambers, to the outside of the entire room, and to the chamber in the center. The walls and doors are made of a polymylar that can be called both reflective and transparent. That is, when looking at a door one can see through the door to the other side and at the same time see one's own reflection in the door.

In each chamber are a number of microphones connected to a delayed recording and playback device and a number of speakers. When I say something in, for example, Chamber One, five seconds later my words are played back over a speaker in Chamber Three. When only one person is in the Riley room, this is a most delightful effect. When a series of the chambers are occupied and the occupants are constantly talking, and opening and closing doors as they go from chamber to chamber, the effect is devastating to normal consciousness and rational functioning. It becomes impossible to tell who said what, where, and when; meanwhile, the interplay between real image and reflection adds to the general quandary.

Riley called the room the "Time-Lag Accumulator," a sonic gallery module.

Further Resources

Riley installed this particular room for an exhibit, decades ago, at New York's Automation House. The original was executed for the Magic Theatre Exhibit in Kansas City and captured in the book *The Magic Theatre* by Ralph Coe. A video of Riley describing "tape loops," a concept he developed with the late Pauline Oliveros, can be found on the *Book of Highs* YouTube playlist. For audio of looping in action, listen to Riley's "Mescalin Mix" and "Music for the Gift" as well as several songs from Brian Eno (a fan of Riley's Time-Lag Accumulator system), who used the approach on "The Heavenly Music Corporation," "Discreet Music," and "Evening Star." All these songs are on the *Book of Highs* Spotify playlist.

225 Binaural beats

An auditory illusion that might alter your brain waves.

You hear two tones extremely close in frequency, one in each ear. Then, a third tone appears. It's not coming from your headphones, it's not coming from your ears. It's coming from the front of your head. Or is it the back? You can't quite place it.

What you are experiencing are the auditory illusions known as binaural beats. These illusions occur when the brain has difficulty processing two tones at frequencies less than 40 Hz apart. The overlap of such frequencies is something that rarely occurs in nature. Binaural beats bridge the difference in the two tones by creating a third tone.

Biophysicist Gerald Oster studied these beats in the 1970s and discovered that they also affected other parts of the body in addition to the auditory illusions created in what we hear. Of late, researchers have been looking into how this third tone might direct one's brain waves toward particular frequencies linked to altered states of consciousness, such as alpha brain waves—associated with relaxation and sleep—which exist between 8 and 14 Hz. By creating a binaural beat in this range, you might drive your brain's electrical activity toward this alpha frequency range. Still others try to create binaural beats in the delta (1–4 Hz) and theta (4–8 Hz) brain wave ranges, often cited as a means of creating ultra-relaxed states and causing some people to quickly fall asleep. More research on these phenomena is needed.

Further Resources

The *Book of Highs* playlist on Spotify features several examples of binaural beats.

· ·

226 Missing frequencies

Your brain can sense what it cannot hear.

W hile your brain creates binaural beats, there are limits to what our hearing can accomplish. Japanese musician Ryoji Ikeda notes that the human hearing range is between 20 Hz and 20 kHz. Even though we can't "hear" frequencies out of this range, his work demonstrates that we can "feel" them and/or sense their absence. As Ikeda describes in the notes for his recent album: "A high frequency sound is used that the listener becomes aware of only upon its disappearance."

Listen—to Ikeda's music, to the world around you. What aren't you hearing? Just because it's not there *to you* doesn't mean it's not there at all. Reality is relative.

Further Resources

I keda's album with "missing" frequencies is titled *+/-*. Play it through to its end, even when you think it's being "silent." You might be surprised when it ends and the true "silence" takes over. His audio-visual installation "Transfinite" can be found on the *Book of Highs* YouTube playlist. (Note the warning about the potential for seizures when watching and listening to this video of sound and light art.)

· ·

227 Infinity room

A beautiful, glowing world that goes on forever.

A n infinity room gives the feeling of being in infinite space. Through an arrangement of glass, thousands of light bulbs, and mirrors, it creates an effect of endlessness. When one steps into an Infinity Room one immediately notices that all the walls, the entire ceiling, and the very floor one is standing on are covered with row after row of amber bulbs. These rows of bulbs, thanks to the invisible arrangement of the mirrors, give the depth impression of continuous backward recession from the wall. That recession never ends. Being in the room gives a feeling of total suspension, total stoppage. The effect is instantaneous. All one's preconceived notions about *real*

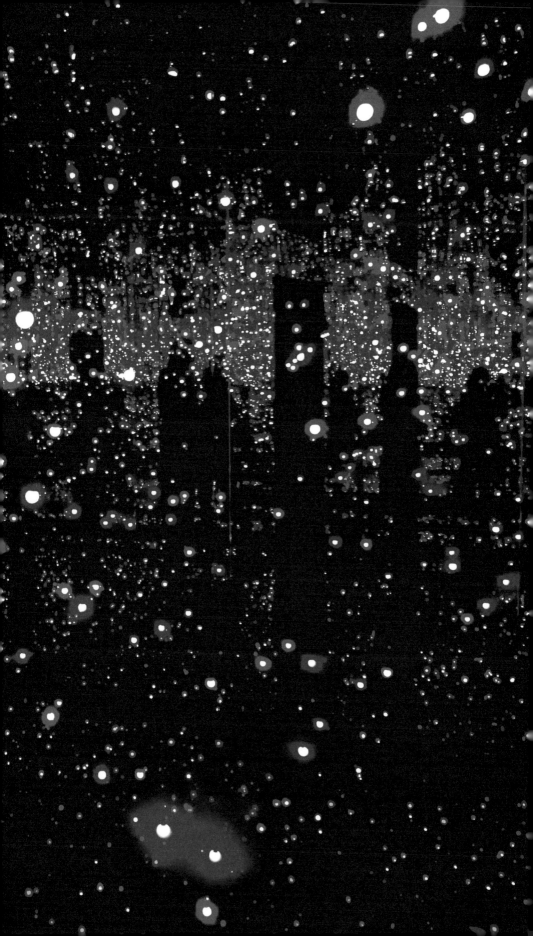

space are left behind, outside the room. This warping of the space sense also affects one's experience of time. With no spatial landmarks and no boundaries, time, too, goes on toward infinity.

A contemporary version of the infinity room concept has been perfected by the Japanese artist Yayoi Kusama. Her most recent exhibit, "Yayoi Kusama: Infinity Mirrors," is touring the United States through 2019.

Further Resources

Videos of both Kusama's modern infinity room and one by Stanley Landesman, an early pioneer in the field, can be viewed on the *Book of Highs* YouTube playlist.

228 Magnets

A forcefield of nature.

Large industrial magnets have tremendously powerful force fields surrounding them. When entering these force fields, one's own systems become greatly affected and the pulls and tugs, seeming to come from out of thin air, are unique and interesting. Be careful not to be wearing or carrying anything that will be torn from you by the magnet's force.

229 Transcranial magnetic stimulation

Many magnetic pulses can change your brain.

Magnets may also be able to change your mood. In transcranial magnetic stimulation (TMS), a large magnetic coil is placed against the scalp near a particular area of the brain linked to mood regulation (the left prefrontal cortex). Magnetic pulses are then sent through the skull to stimulate nerve cells and potentially activate regions of the brain that have decreased in those with depression (by stimulating mood-boosting neurotransmitters like serotonin and dopamine). It's given without anesthesia and the patient is alert the whole time. Typically, a forty-minute session is given daily, for up to six weeks.

Further Resources

Although research is still ongoing, there have been many studies on the effects of TMS. See "A Practical Guide to Diagnostic Transcranial Magnetic Stimulation: Report of an IFCN Committee" (2012) and "Evidence-Based Guidelines on the Therapeutic Use of Repetitive Transcranial Magnetic Stimulation (rTMS)," both in the journal *Clinical Neurophysiology,* or "Daily Left Prefrontal Repetitive Transcranial Magnetic Stimulation for Acute Treatment of Medication-Resistant Depression," in the *American Journal of Psychiatry* (2011) to start.

• •

230 Negative ionization

How a charged atmosphere can charge you.

Our atmosphere is constantly being ionized. Cosmic rays, radioactive soil elements, ultraviolet radiation, thunderstorms, winds, and the friction of blowing dust and particulate matter cause ions in the atmosphere to be positively or negatively charged.

Positive ionization is heaviest in urban areas. Negative ionization is most prevalent in the desert, on the open seas, at the tops of mountains, and in any spot where a thunderstorm has just occurred. Positive ions make the air feel stale, and cause fatigue and depression. Negative ions give feelings of alertness and mild excitation.

It is surmised by researchers on negative ionization that their presence in the bloodstream enables more oxygen to reach our cells and tissues and allows it to get there quicker. Positive ionization has the opposite effect.

Further Resources

Philip K. Dick's novel *Ubik* has part of its plot centered around the effects of negative ionization.

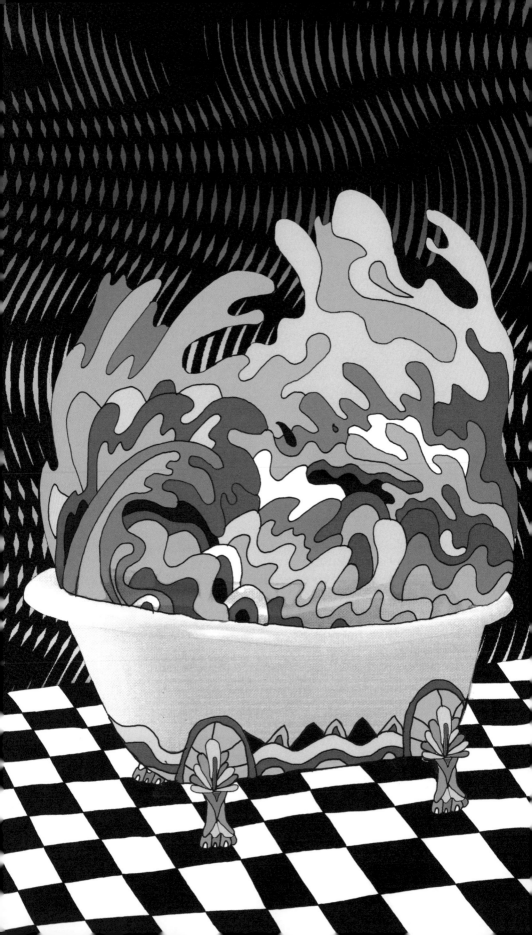

231 Psychedelic bathtub

When moiré patterns, lights, and a luminescent bubble bath make a bathroom like no other.

Harry Hermon, a researcher into psychedelics and altered states of consciousness, developed a psychedelic bathtub that might more properly be called a psychedelic bathroom. The room where the bathtub is located is fitted with a variety of light-and-sound fixtures, including a revolving mirrored ball with spots, color wheels, and strobes. On the walls are a number of mounted moving moiré patterns (see No. 232), and other colored lights that may be varied as to intensity and operation.

The subject is told to undress and run their bath. While the bath is running, a luminescent bubble bath is added to the water.

When the bath is drawn, the subject gets in and relaxes. Then the lights start to move, the moiré patterns begin shimmering and revolving, the strobes flicker at a variety of different speeds, the mirrored ball sends beams of rainbow light shooting across the room, and all of the above reflect and shine onto and through the multicolored soap bubbles. When sounds—chants, electronic music, or random noise patterns—are added, the bathroom becomes a fantastic room, and the subject becomes high.

With a little effort, the purchase of the correct equipment, and the proper design implementations, the psychedelic bathtub can be assembled almost anywhere.

232 Moiré patterns

Ancient optical art.

Moiré patterns are everywhere in our environment. The easiest way to see one is to take two identical black pocket combs, align them, and then move one back and forth. The patterns made by each comb's teeth will combine to give an impression of a third and moving pattern.

We also see moiré patterns on the highway as we drive. Two different types of fencing or two different sets of posts will create the same effect as the pocket combs do, with the automobile supplying the movement.

Moiré, or watered silk, was invented by the Chinese. The moiré pattern sensation can be stimulated by many other patterns, such as those presented by optical art.

One of the more ingenious uses for these patterns is to mount them on a wall attached to a vibrating and/or rotating device. Though moiré patterns do not always have to move to produce their hallucinatory effects, when they do move these effects are greatly heightened.

233 Seeing your eye

A DIY project that allows you to see the intricacy and beauty of your own eye.

The late biophysicist Gerald Oster showed how to see the internal structure of the eye and the eyelid. Take a length of fiber optics light pipe (available via multiple sources online) and place one end on the lens of a very powerful source of light (e.g., a high-intensity reading light). Put the other end of the light pipe on the lid of your closed eye. You will have to move around the end that is on your eyelid, since the eye never focuses on any one place for very long. What you will see as you move it around is a show of internal cinema that rivals the best hallucinations: the structure of the circulatory system of the eyelid and part of the system of nerves, veins, and arteries of the eye itself.

234 Electrical stimulation of the mastoid

Low-frequency stimulation of the bone behind your ear creates the sensation of spinning.

When NASA was trying to determine what to do to ease the feelings of nausea that astronauts who are in a spinning, tumbling capsule experience, they considered the production of countersensations to mask the effect. One of the experiments was the generation of an electrical charge to the astronauts' mastoids (the bone behind the ear), which, when controlled properly, would give them the sensation of spinning in the opposite direction. This would have neutralized any spinning or tumbling effects.

This idea was abandoned and retro-rockets were finally adopted to deal with the problem. Gerald Oster picked up his idea from NASA's research. In his lab, he hooked people up to an audio generator and produced low-voltage, low-frequency stimulation to the mastoid. This stimulation was phased to create a beat, generating a third sensation made by the proper phasing of two different frequencies. (Beat is also the basis of moiré patterns.) At eight thousand cycles or more the subject felt the room beginning to spin in one direction. When the phasing was reversed and the tuning slowed, the subject experienced the room spinning in the opposite direction.

Don't try this at home!

More recently, this kind of stimulation has been used in conjunction with medical treatments for patients suffering from tinnitus, migraine frequency, ischemic stroke, and other maladies.

Further Resources

A recent study on the use of mastoid stimulation for this purpose, "Ultrasonic Bone Stimulation: Countermeasure to Orthostatic Intolerance," was conducted by Chester A. Ray of Penn State University from 2004 to 2006.

· ·

235 Electric clothing

When your body becomes light.

E lectric clothing was introduced by fashion designer Diana Dew in the late 1960s. Wearing a dress of her own design and making, she appeared as a walking, bleeping, flashing body. Her dress was wired to a battery worn around her waist. The eye delighted as different parts of her dress lit up, flashed, changed color.

The development of LED lighting systems has exploded electric clothing in the twenty-first century. As computing technology has been miniaturized, it has enabled clothing not just to feature lighting but to incorporate many other kinds of displays. Some of these computing elements have even been incorporated into the fabric. Thanks to rapid advancements in computer-augmented electric clothing, we can now become walking displays, showing virtually anything we wish through our apparel. We can be walking,

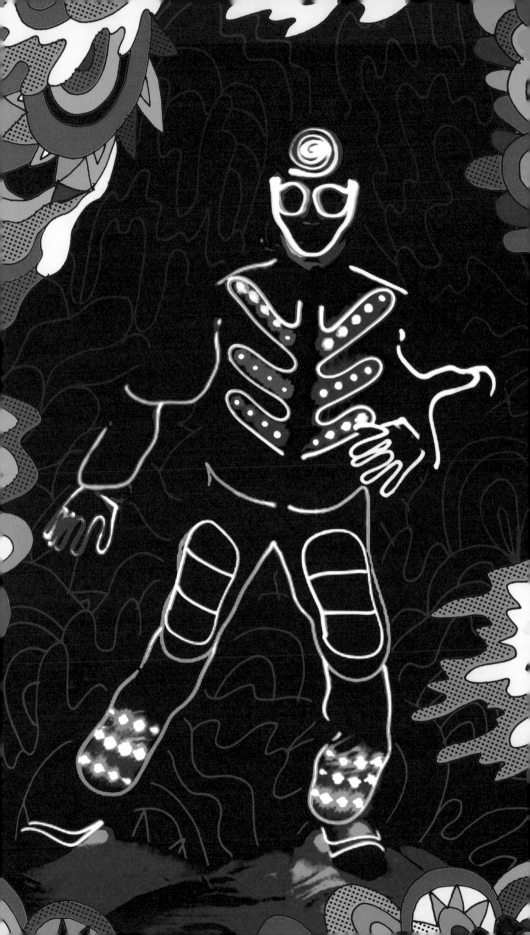

standing, even seated art exhibits, showing any imagery on our clothing that can be displayed on a computer screen, tablet, or smartphone.

Further Resources

A selection from Tom Hyman's profile of Diana Dew and her electric clothing appears in Marshall McLuhan and Quentin Fiore's *War and Peace in the Global Village*. Electric clothing is usually custom made but can also be acquired from scores of manufacturers; it can be found with a simple web search.

· ·

236 Ganzfeld effect

Prolonged exposure to a featureless field can have extraordinary effects.

"Ganzfeld," German for "total or complete field," is a form of perceptual and sensory deprivation. The Ganzfeld effect—analogous to prisoner's cinema, audio repetition, and other forms of sense dep—can be experienced in any environment with a "featureless" visual field, like the pitch black of a cave or the endless white of the Arctic.

In the experiments that took place in the 1930s, it was noted that, when subjects stared at a field of vision without any features, they not only saw visions but measurements of their brain waves showed corresponding alterations.

But you don't have to venture to the Arctic to experience this unique state. Here are a few steps to create your own "total field" at home.

1 Establish visual deprivation. Use a sleeping mask or two halves of a ping-pong ball (one half for each eye) to cover your eyes.

2 Create a "total field." You still might see light/background beyond this covering, so you will also need to make sure you're in front of a blank field. Visit the *Book of Highs* YouTube playlist and select the Ganzfeld effect video. Make sure it is occupying the full screen of your device.

3 Establish auditory deprivation. The video will include white noise. Be sure to wear headphones to block out all other sounds. If you'd like to also play binaural beats (available on the *Book of Highs* Spotify playlist), they can heighten the experience.

4 Sit down. With your eyes covered and your headphones in place, play the video for thirty minutes. When it ends, remove your headphones and mask. What do you see, hear, and feel in the world around you?

. . . .

237 Electrosleep

Hacking your brain waves to encourage sleep.

Electrosleep, or Russian sleep as it is often called, refers to the use of electrical machines that enable people to live with less sleep than they would normally require. Electrosleep involves the direct manipulation of the electrical charge and power of human brain waves. This manipulation is accomplished by machines that are available in the United States only to those who meet government research qualifications.

The sleep machine sends out an electrical current through electrodes that are attached to the subject's temples and forehead. The current occurs at specific frequencies meant to stimulate the brain to produce serotonin and other neurochemicals that cause sleep. Treatment usually lasts for a half hour.

Research has so far been applied to people suffering from insomnia, anxiety, depression, and drug addiction. The machine is used to help them relax so that they can get to sleep without the aid of medication.

Further Resources

The medical technology company Fisher Wallace makes an electrosleep machine. You need a prescription from your healthcare provider (it is prescribed for depression and insomnia). See their website (fisherwallace .com) for details on the machine and how to obtain one.

. . . .

238 Sound and motion sensors

Devices that increase bodily awareness.

Motion sensors may be attached to you (or to anything else you'd like) and will report, by way of an auditory feedback signal, whenever motion occurs. This helps you to keep still, and also increases your awareness of how often you move without knowing it.

Sound sensors work on the same principle. Connect them to whatever you would like to monitor; anytime a sound is created, you will be informed by a beep, or a buzz, or a light. They can be used to increase your awareness of what true silence is.

239 Electronically generated visual illusions

Projects to create illusions in your own home.

In No. 28, the nature of culturally based visual illusions is discussed. Here I will describe some devices that generate illusions.

One device is an ordinary desk lamp fitted with an opaque shade and an on/off switch that can be operated every second. Seat yourself so that you are about eighteen inches away from the lamp and gaze at the area on the surface of the desk under the lamp. Begin to switch the lamp on and off about once every second. After a dozen on/offs, a small disk of light will appear, just below the bulb, whenever the lamp is turned on. When turned off, a shadow, circular in form, will sweep across the field of vision, and the light will contract into a disk and fade away.

If you place a complex, rich pattern on a turntable and operate the turntable under bright illumination at 78 rpm, the black sections of the drawing will become slightly purple. Reduce the speed to 45 rpm and a yellow haze will appear. At 33 rpm, most color perception will recede.

The combination of a variety of op art patterns and a turntable or other spinning device can produce very powerful and effective visual illusions.

Further Resources

Both of Richard Gregory's books *Eye and Brain* and *The Intelligent Eye,* as well as his book *Visual Illusions,* will give you a lot of ideas.

240 OKPLD

How a simple project with light, poster board, and a turntable can enhance your perceptions.

OKPLD stands for the Optokinetic Perceptual Learning Device for Sensory Stimulation and Learning. The device was developed by Eleanor Criswell while she was working toward her doctorate at the University of Florida in 1970. You can make your own OKPLD at home. You need black poster board, strips of newspaper (just black and white—no color), a high-intensity light, and a turntable.

Using the poster board, make a paper drum six inches high and eight inches in diameter. Cut newspaper into strips and attach them to the drum's vertical sides. Then place the drum on a three-speed turntable.

Sit facing the OKPLD so that your gaze falls on one side of the drum, watching with an intent but relaxed gaze. The drum should be revolved at 33⅓ rpm for three to five minutes. During this time, watch the design; it is best to count while watching. Criswell suggests that you say: 1—1 AM, 2—1 AM, 3—1 AM, etc., through 10 and back to 1 again.

While you are watching the revolving drum, the light is illuminating the area, and you are enhancing your perceptions for the rest of the day. You should have a timer nearby to make sure you keep viewing for about five minutes. At the completion of a viewing, when the turntable and the drum stop, a motion aftereffect will be manifest for a brief period of time.

This effect and the enhancement of sensory awareness are the most frequently reported alterations of consciousness achieved by the OKPLD.

· ·

241 Repetition tapes

When the recording stays the same, but what you hear changes.

Repetition tapes were discovered by R. L. Gregory of England and Richard Warren of the United States. A repetition tape is a loop tape that repeats, exactly, the same sound, word, or phrase over and over again, indefinitely.

My first exposure to them was through John Lilly. Lilly played a tape with the word "COGITATE" repeating over and over to a roomful of more than a hundred people. Everyone heard the tape change into another word. My own experience was of being able to let the word change into other words, but of always being able to return to the initial perception: that of hearing "COGITATE." After about eight minutes of listening I became tense and nervous; I was tired of listening to the same word repeated over and over. Suddenly, the tape changed. It said "MELT INTO IT." I could not return to "COGITATE" totally for another minute. Then I heard nothing but "COGITATE" until Lilly turned the tape machine off, after some ten minutes. I turned to a friend to compare notes.

"Tape changed, didn't it?" I said.

"It sure did," said my friend. "Count to ten."

"What?" I said in disbelief.

"The tape changed from saying 'COGITATE' to saying 'COUNT TO TEN.' I heard it change. It wasn't me."

Everyone in the room heard it change to a different word or phrase. However, the tape *never* changed. It always said "COGITATE."

Lilly reports that almost all people's brains will function this way in order to cope with a boring, unchanging, repetitious input. The only people who have never heard such tapes change are the congenitally blind. It is thought that this is because of their need to correctly perceive auditory cues in their environment. The sighted can afford auditory hallucinations.

Further Resources

The origin of repetition tapes is discussed in Nigel Calder's *The Mind of Man*. Lilly's COGITATE repetition tape is available on the *Book of Highs* YouTube playlist.

242–245
BIOFEEDBACK

How technology is changing our awareness and control of our bodies and minds.

Feedback is information. When a process is being performed and the resulting knowledge of the process is made accessible to the performer, then feedback takes place. Feedback involves a knowledge of certain results being reintegrated into a system.

Biofeedback is a new frontier in research and creativity, combining the activities of consciousness, psychology, philosophy, electronics, and physiology. What biofeedback does is apply feedback technology to internal, visceral systems. These systems are usually out of our conscious, voluntary control. Biofeedback brings internal functions out into the area of consciousness, and thereby allows learning and control to take place.

Applications of this method hold great promise for the treatment of illness and for use in rehabilitation. Great excitement has also been generated because of the possibility of its use in altering states of consciousness.

For centuries, select groups of men have known that it is possible to become aware of, and control, internal states. Yogis in India, Tibet, and elsewhere can speed up and slow down breathing, heartbeat and pulse, and blood circulation, as well as control other functions. The Yogi Swami Rama came to the United States in the 1960s to demonstrate some of his awesome abilities of psychophysiological control. One astounding demonstration was that of his ability to control the temperature of his hands; he could, within two minutes, raise the temperature on one part of his hand ten degrees higher than the temperature on another part of the same hand, some two inches away! This Yogi was tested by Elmer and Alyce Green of the Menninger Foundation, people who pioneered the study of voluntary control of internal states.

In many ways, biofeedback mimics Yogis' experiences in training. A Yogi spends years learning how to zero in his consciousness on a physiological indicator, say, the heartbeat. After learning to become aware of his heartbeat, he can then learn to use this awareness to control the way in which his heart beats. Biofeedback works much the same way, in that the subject can be connected to a feedback device, an EKG (electrocardiograph), for information about his heart. When he can measure and compare, internally, the states that are being reported by the feedback device, the next step will be to use that feedback information to control the state being reported. If his heart beats too slowly, he can speed it up; if it beats too quickly, he can slow it down. Yogis take years to learn this kind of awareness and control. Technological instrumentation now allows this kind of learning to be acquired in a matter of months, even days.

Feedback learning and control work is now being conducted in a variety of research areas described on the following pages.

Further Resources

For resources, events, and therapists who utilize biofeedback, consult the Association for Applied Psychophysiology and Biofeedback (aapb.org), the Biofeedback Certification International Alliance (bcia.org), and the International Society for Neurofeedback and Research (isnr.org). To stay abreast of developments and events within the consciousness hacking movement, visit its website (cohack.life). For informative overviews of the intersection between altered states and biofeedback, including those who support and criticize them, see "Meditation and neurofeedback" in the journal *Frontiers in Psychology* (October 7, 2013) and the U.S. military's National Center for Telehealth & Technology (t2health.dcoe.mil). The 2010 study on neurofeedback and neuroplasticity was published in the *European Journal of Neuroscience* under the title "Endogenous control of waking brain rhythms induces neuroplasticity in humans by Tomas Ros et al. (2010). More information on the devices mentioned here can be found on their respective websites.

242 Brain-wave biofeedback

The electricity of the mind.

U sing electroencephalographic devices, subjects are taught to control and manipulate their own brain waves. This research was initiated in the United States by Joe Kamiya. Most of the work in brain-wave feedback has centered on one particular brain wave, alpha. (There are four main varieties of brain waves: *Beta,* with a frequency ranging from 14 to 50 cycles per second; *Alpha,* with a frequency ranging from 8 to 13 cycles per second; *Theta,* with a frequency ranging from 4 to 7 cycles per second; and *Delta,* with a frequency ranging from 0.5 to 3.5 cycles per second. Beta indicates mental and visual activity. Alpha is present during relaxation and some dream states. Theta is sometimes present in dream and other sleep states as well as in some relaxed waking states. Delta is indicative of deep sleep.)

Subjects were trained with EEGs (electroencephalograms) or the like by being given a feedback indication of when they were producing alpha. Subjects learned quickly and most could generate alpha at will after several hours of intensive training. Studies of the EEG states present in meditating Zen masters and monks, and in Yogis, indicated that alpha, and some related theta states, were the results of the years spent in meditative practice.

As research has continued, experimenters have become interested in a borderline area between alpha and theta, an area identified by brain waves ranging from 6 to 9 cycles per second, with amplitudes of more than 50 microvolts. (Most brain waves produce power in the range below 25 microvolts.) Several experiments are now being conducted to establish a link between creativity, ESP, and other factors and this borderline brain-wave area.

What must be stressed with reference to the future of brain-wave feedback is that all studies, formal or informal, professional or nonprofessional, are being pursued in an area of relative ignorance. Though subjects can now learn to generate alpha and other brain-wave patterns at will, in short periods of time, and though the resultant states of consciousness are described with adjectives ranging from relaxing to psychedelic, most researchers indicate that the field is currently in its infancy. No one is yet sure what the difference is between alpha generated from the left cerebral hemisphere and that emanating from the right cerebral hemisphere.

Recent studies in brain implantation and ESB (electrical stimulation of the brain) indicate that alpha itself is generated from within the septum, deep inside the brain. All EEG measurements, by both professional and amateur equipment, are taken from outside the skull. The ability to place electrodes intracerebrally will probably usher in the second, third, or fourth generation of brain-wave–feedback research.

A number of centers have appeared throughout the country, usually supported by the pseudo-scientific research of self-professed psychologists (with and without degrees), that claim to train individuals in controlling brain-wave states without the use of feedback instruments. Usually they quote Joe Kamiya and other authorities out of context and without permission to support their claims. They all have thousands of successful graduates. Their courses cost hundreds and sometimes thousands of dollars. The basis of these courses almost always centers around a mild form of hypnotic induction. Be wary of the smooth-talking salesmen who are now "brain-wave teachers."

243 Electrodermal activity
The electricity of your skin.

Electrodermal activity (EDA) measures the changes in electrical characteristics of the skin. An earlier version of this kind of measurement was the galvanic skin response (GSR).

The main uses for EDA in psychology and psychiatry focus on measuring stress responses and how states like anxiety are handled. When someone in psychotherapy, or undergoing other related mental health assessments and treatments, is asked to recall a traumatic or disturbing experience, measures like EDA, heart rate monitoring, blood pressure and respiratory rate, all autonomically dependent variables, can indicate the subject's state of being in ways that may not be reflected in verbal reports, facial expressions, posture, and the like. In addition, EDA is often used to measure the depth of hypnotic trance.

An example: When a subject was having EDA monitored, a feedback mechanism of a sound was in use. To begin, the feedback mechanism was producing a loud but low whine. A person said to the subject: "What if I were to hit you in the stomach right now?" He made no motion to strike, but, as the subject considered these words, the whine increased in intensity and pitch until it was a piercing howl. As they talked and the subject discovered that the other person had no intention of hitting him, the feedback sounds returned to their original low whine.

••

244 Muscle biofeedback

The electricity of your muscles.

Electromyographic (EMG) feedback is used here to describe work being done using muscle feedback to control tension states. The subject is connected to an EMG device and hears a tone that varies according to the electrical activity present in the muscle or muscles wired for feedback. When we are aroused in exercise, fright, flight, or anxiety, we take on a high degree of muscle tension. Even when not in these states, during waking hours most people have a high degree of muscle tension. If that tension can be drastically reduced, as it can by EMG feedback, then a relaxed and sometimes altered state of consciousness ensues. More often, EMG is used to assess symptoms and investigate possible disease states. The Mayo Clinic indicates that doctors use EMG measurements for more information about the presence of the following symptoms of potential disorders: tingling, numbness, muscle weakness, muscle pain and cramping, and limb pains.

••

245 Heartbeat and respiration biofeedback

The electricity of your heart and breath.

Through the use of feedback coupled with an electrocardiogram (EKG), people have been learning to control their hearts, to make them go faster and slower, to make them beat more evenly and regularly, and to detect any changes in operation. Blood-pressure feedback, through the use of a blood-pressure cuff, has enabled people with high and low blood pressure not only to change their blood pressures, but at the same time to become aware of the states that raise or lower these pressures to begin with. Breath bags, mirrors, and other devices have been used to show a subject the workings of their breathing mechanisms.

Some researchers have been working in areas that include voluntary control learned through feedback of temperature, both for the entire body

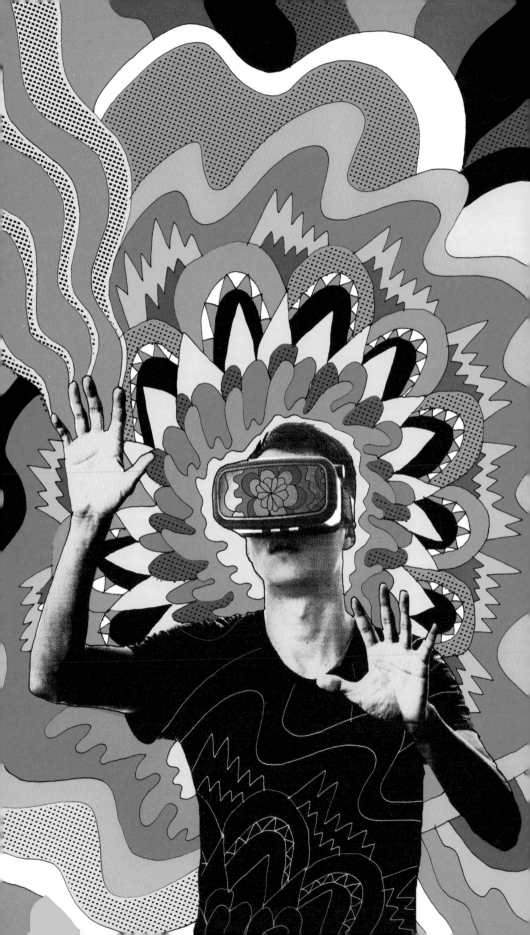

and for separate parts of the body: sweat-gland activity, eye movements, etc. The Greens trained their subjects to control three major neuroanatomical regions: craniospinal, autonomic, and central.

Certainly, the future of biofeedback lies in this area of feedback training and control in combination. To isolate just EEG, EMG, or blood pressure will not bring anywhere near as dramatic results as learned voluntary control in all three states.

• •

246 Virtual reality
Tech that transports us to different worlds.

Virtual reality (VR) is a computer-created set of experiences based in the perception of a contained visual and auditory environment. This is usually done by wearing googles and headphones, or a specific device such as an Oculus Rift, a Samsung Gear, a Google Cardboard, or Google Daydream, and a plethora of other VR devices on the market.* Projected onto the field of vision and enhanced by auditory effects, a virtual environment is created. To the person wearing the headgear, the new environment appears as "reality" because VR systems allow the user to see what it is like to move around and experience different perspectives as generated by the movement of their head and other body parts.

What happens in VR is similar to what pilots and others experience using sophisticated flight and other simulators, replete with visual, auditory, and often motion effects so real that they feel like they're really flying or moving, even though they're not. Putting on a VR device transports the user into a complete world, one full of specific detail and many kinds of effects. Most startling is the sensation of motion and spatial dimensions—as the user moves her head to look one way or the other, the entire world view changes according to her movements. The sensation of being completely enveloped in a new, fantastically rendered environment is overwhelming and at times very disconcerting. Balance can become an issue and nausea can be a most unwelcome side effect.

The new sense of orientation can also cause feelings of displacement and fear, often leading to an unwelcomed altered state of awareness. *Where am I? What is real? How far can I go and what can I really do here? Is that really a cliff edge and dare I walk too close to it. I know it's not real, but . . .*

VR experiences vary widely and wildly. What can be seen on a Google or Samsung device for a mobile phone may, depending on the software/content, be inferior to or superior to what can be discovered in VR research and development labs; more typically, though, it won't be as good.

Further, a newer form of VR, called mixed reality (MR) combines aspects of VR with AR (augmented reality). This mixture can enable the user to interact, often with tactile feedback, with what are real objects in the real world or are only virtual objects that seem to be real objects in the environment. The user can pick up a book, open it, turn the pages, and read the text. Or, as many experienced recently, users can chase down Pokémons in Pokémon Go games.

Included here are a few examples of VR experiences that might alter one's consciousness. These are some of the leading programs as of this writing; no doubt, there will be plenty of exciting additions in the future.

- "When We Die," designed by Dana Abrassart, Leslie Ruckman, and Paula Ceballos, offers a guided meditation focused on the contemplation of mortality.

- "Chi": Tim Gallati, founder of the Harvard Divinity School's Virtual Reality Group, designed, along with fellow students, "Chi," a VR program that uses tactile feedback and visual cues to teach Tai Chi.

- "Guided Meditation VR" offers nine guided sessions, immersing you in different relaxing settings, incorporating visuals, music, and biofeedback (a heart rate monitor) to better enhance your meditative experience.

- "MicrodoseVR" is a kaleidoscopic journey by Android Jones, an artist who does a lot of VR/animation work, especially for events like Burning Man.

Further Resources

Note that the field of VR changes quickly in the resources and experiences it will be capable of offering. Tomorrow's VR may look, sound, and feel far different from today's. Some current resources: "Can Virtual Meditation Help You Hack Your Consciousness?" in the *Village Voice* (October 5, 2016). There are two great episodes from the podcast *Buddhist Geeks* on the pros and the cons of using VR as "contemplative technology." Both episodes, "Virtual Reality IRL" and "Virtual Reality and the Tea Ceremony," are available on SoundCloud. You can learn more about the programs mentioned here on their respective websites (guidedmeditationvr.com, whenwedievr.com, microdosevr.com, and on Vimeo for "Chi").

247 Augmented reality

Adding to the way we see the world.

Augmented reality (AR) first came to our attention through the not fully successful experiment of Google Glass, a headset, worn like glasses, that superimposed computer-generated materials onto the user's field of vision. Before Google Glass, earlier versions of AR were mostly for guide purposes—either in travel or art—superimposing relevant information onto a field of view. Now, as of this writing, Apple and other major players in the computing world are devising more advanced AR systems, hoping for better results and an acceptance by the consumer marketplace that was not forthcoming for Google Glass.

It seems that AR could certainly lead to new and different kinds of experiences as we visit museums and other venues where augmented information can help to provide useful information, facts, directions, etc., and, potentially, even mind-altering experiences.

However, a warning is in order: As our devices, like mobile phones and home assistants (Amazon Alexa/Dot, Google Home, Apple HomePod, etc.) become smarter they will also become smarter about who we are, where we are, what we're doing and they may even be able to make good guesses about what we may want and what we may want to do next. In the future, when I walk into a room, will my smartphone automatically link up with other screens in that room? If I'm wearing an AR device and I look at something in a store, can another merchant see what I'm looking at and make me a better offer? The shrinking world of personal privacy may well be even more up for grabs, to the highest bidder, in the future. Caveat emptor.

248 Mutual wave machine

An audio-visual capsule that allows two people to truly sync up.

Is it possible to truly be on the same wavelength as another person? A mutual wave machine (MWM) is a small environment, usually a capsule that seats two people and attempts to do just that. The equipment inside enables the pair to synchronize their brain waves, heart rates, and breathing. Creators Suzanne Dikker and Siena Oristaglio describe the experiences to be found in their MWM this way:

> Enclosed by an intimate capsule and immersed in an audiovisual environment that responds and reflects their shared brain activity, two visitors can directly experience and manipulate their internal efforts to approach each other, or distance themselves from each other.
>
> During the experience, greater brain-wave synchronization is reflected in greater vividness and more coherent and recognizable audiovisual patterns, while lack of synchronization strays towards dark audio-visual chaos: a faint ringing in the ears and static in the retinas. The audience can hear and observe the internal dance unfold through the semi-translucent shell of the Machine.

Further Resources

See Suzanne Dikker's website focusing on her mutual wave machine projects (suzannedikker.net). Another of her MWM projects can be seen at Marina Abramovíc Institute (mai.art), along with a short film of the device.

• •

249 Holophonic sound

Hearing recordings in three dimensions can produce tactile, otherworldly sensations.

In the 1980s, Argentine researcher Hugo Zuccarelli developed a recording technique that made recorded samples sound three-dimensional. As a result, we hear the recorded sound so realistically that it can stimulate our other senses. For instance, a recording that re-creates a haircut will cause listeners to feel the snips of the scissors, the buzz of the razor beneath their ear.

Even though you know the sounds are coming from your headphones, it will feel like they are moving behind you and in front of you.

Further Resources

The haircut recording is available on the *Book of Highs* YouTube playlist.

250 Simulated body illusions

Out-of-body experiences through technology.

N eurologically, out-of-body experiences (see No. 60) are a form of bodily illusion arising from a disruption of our visual and proprioceptive (sense of body position) systems. An OBE creates an altered state by disrupting the seemingly reliable constant: our sense of "self." You know your body is your own because you can feel it, because you look at the world from its perspective. But what if that changed?

Swedish researcher Henrik Ehrsson uses technology to manipulate your brain's visual, touch, and proprioceptive sensations to create feelings of switching bodies with a doll or watching your own body from across the room. When neurologist and author Oliver Sacks tried some of the experiments at Ehrsson's lab, he was convinced he had grown a third arm.

In addition to creating an astonishing altered state, Ehrsson's research has many practical applications, such as eliminating "phantom limb" pain from prosthetics by assigning the artificial limb visual feedback.

Here are two of Ehrsson's simulated OBE experiments:

The Out-of-Body Illusion

At Ehrsson's lab, the subject wears a VR headset that shows him a view from a camera directed at his back. Using two rods, the researcher simultaneously touches the subject's chest and moves the other rod toward the camera lens. For the subject, the combination of seeing a hand moving toward the camera as he feels his chest getting prodded and seeing his body from behind on the headset creates a sense that his body is floating behind the one he sees.

The Barbie Doll Illusion

Another Ehrsson experiment: The subject here wears a headset video display that allows him to see from the perspective of a doll. As in the rubber hand experiment discussed below, the researcher strokes the subject's body and doll's body simultaneously in the same locations, and the subject interprets the felt touches to be caused by the rod that he sees touching the doll. The subject is then shown a cube and asked to show the size of the cube with their hands. If the illusion works, they will overestimate the size of the cube, as the perspective of the doll's tiny body causes the world to appear gigantic.

Try your own body illusion. In the 1990s, American researchers devised the "Rubber Hand Illusion," which caused subjects to believe that a rubber hand was their own. Since you don't need high-tech equipment, you can try this at home.

You'll need: An inflated rubber glove, a piece of cardboard, and two paintbrushes.

Place the fake hand on a table in front of you and place your real hand out of view behind the cardboard. Ask a friend to stroke the fake hand and your real one simultaneously with the paintbrushes. Watch only the fake hand. Soon enough, you will start to see it as your own. For an added thrill: Have your friend slam the fake hand with a hammer—you'll certainly get a scare!

Further Resources

See the work of Henrik Ehrsson at the Karolinska Institute in Sweden (ehrssonlab.se). *Hallucinations* by Oliver Sacks also describes the many incredible instances of such simulated and nondrug hallucinogenic experiences. Videos of the rubber hand illusion and Ehrsson's OBE experiments are available on the *Book of Highs* YouTube playlist.

• •

251 Autonomous sensory meridian response

A sound-stimulated tingling sensation experienced by the lucky few.

Autonomous sensory meridian response (ASMR) is an experience of mysterious sensations—a tingling feeling, a sensing of static electricity, something akin to being scratched—that typically begins on the scalp and moves down the back of the neck toward the upper spine. It is brought about by certain sounds, including crinkling, squishing, whispering, or the soft sounds associated with a mundane, repetitive task (e.g., a routine, painless exam or questionnaire, turning pages.). There are many ASMR videos, mostly on YouTube, posted of people whispering and giving soothing instructions to induce these experiences, by people who refer to themselves as ASMRtists.

Further Resources

Visit the *Book of Highs* YouTube playlist for examples of ASMR videos. In *The Atlantic*'s December 2013 article "How to Have a Brain Orgasm," the author notes that people sometimes have ASMR experiences when getting a haircut or an ear exam: "The strongest tingle feels like sparkles or little fireworks, and gives you the feeling of being pleasantly exhausted." Another article, in the *Guardian,* "ASMR and 'Head Orgasms': What's the Science Behind It?" includes further explorations into the ASMR phenomenon.

• •

252 Video games

A challenge, a pleasure, a new frontier.

"Video games" as a term has come to designate any number of games that are played on electronic devices, especially those with displays. With revenues approaching $100 billion each year, they are the third largest branch of entertainment in the United States, behind broadcast and cable television. But it is what happens when people play video games that is so special. These mostly three-dimensional depictions of complicated, complex, and often aesthetically pleasing environments are engaging, engrossing, and more, ushering users into worlds that often become of their own making: radiant play to the players.

In order to better understand the true nature of video games and altered states of awareness, I consulted my son, Zachary (b. 1990), a game player for at least two decades. He cited the different worlds that games make it possible for the player to enter into and interact with: Oftentimes, great stories and characters abound. In TV and movies, you root for or against the main characters; in video games, most often, you are the main character and, often, the aim of the game is to survive challenging and threatening circumstances you encounter.

In addition, in some games, like *Skyrim* and *Fallout,* even in *World of Warcraft,* you are also responsible for the care and well-being of family members and others you care about, as well as your common homestead, which in some games you construct, maintain, and expand. You become the game when playing and, as Zach notes, this can induce altered states of awareness, focus, and experience. And, as he warns, playing these games can become addictive.

Further Resources

Video games can alter consciousness and perspectives. Two recent examples in a rapidly changing and developing, high powered field: *Soundself,* a trance-inducing game created by Robin Arnoff, and *Ambient Flight,* a game that allows you to see the world from the sky, as if you were a bird.

• •

253 Brain music

Hearing your brain waves at work.

Using a brain-wave feedback device, David Rosenboom let his own brain waves determine the kind of music he would make. This concert/experiment occurred in December 1970. It was the first public demonstration of the use of brain-wave feedback to produce an art form. Rosenboom links his brain waves to an input device of his own musical synthesizer, the Neurona.

Further Resources

Rosenboom gave his performance at Automation House. He holds the Richard Seaver Distinguished Chair in Music in The Herb Alpert School of Music at California Institute of the Arts, where he has been dean of the School of Music since 1990. Current information about his activities can be found on his website (davidrosenboom.com). Listen to his brain-wave–generated song "Invisible Gold and Philosophers' Stones" on the *Book of Highs* Spotify playlist.

254 Electrical stimulation of the brain

Charge your mind.

E lectrical stimulation of the brain (ESB) is, along with biofeedback, the area with the greatest potential for future control, understanding, and expansion of consciousness. ESB is now being used in two major ways. One, to investigate the actual makeup and operation of the brain. Two, for therapeutic purposes.

As noted above, measuring the brain's spontaneous electrical activity by means of surface electrodes (EEG) does not reflect the actual activity of the brain. A new procedure is now being developed and tested that will be able to tell us where specific types of cerebral activity initiate from and how they function. This method involves the surgical implantation of the intracerebral electrodes which will monitor electrical activity at source points. Taking a reading of electrical brain activity from the temples or the occipital is quite different from taking a reading from within the brain septum. Knowledge of the actual location of the brain's different centers will speed conscious control over brain usage, much in the same way the brain-wave feedback enables rapid learning of control over reported brain-wave activity.

The newest approach to ESB will take a more computer-augmented approach by, in some applications, placing computer chips and processors into the body and the brain.

Here again, don't try this at home—yet!

255 Living

The most precious state.

Index

· ·

About the Author

EDWARD ROSENFELD is a writer and editor. His newsletter, INTELLIGENCE (1984–2017) was the first to cover the history and development of neural networks and artificial intelligence. His three books on neural nets include *Talking Nets: An Oral History of Neural Networks*. He also wrote *An Oral History of Gestalt Therapy*. He was a founding editor of *Omni* magazine as well as an intellectual property executive at Columbia University. His screenplay, *MKULTRA*, has been adapted for the opera as *Huxley's Last Trip*. His new website is worldworking.net. He was born and still lives in New York City.